Kélvia Coelho Campos Paula
Zélia Maria de Sousa A. Santos
Zélia M. S. A. Santos

Nursing Consultation

Kélvia Coelho Campos Paula
Zélia Maria de Sousa A. Santos
Zélia M. S. A. Santos

Nursing Consultation

Self-care for people with hypertension

ScienciaScripts

Imprint

Any brand names and product names mentioned in this book are subject to trademark, brand or patent protection and are trademarks or registered trademarks of their respective holders. The use of brand names, product names, common names, trade names, product descriptions etc. even without a particular marking in this work is in no way to be construed to mean that such names may be regarded as unrestricted in respect of trademark and brand protection legislation and could thus be used by anyone.

Cover image: www.ingimage.com

This book is a translation from the original published under ISBN 978-613-9-72730-8.

Publisher:
Sciencia Scripts
is a trademark of
Dodo Books Indian Ocean Ltd. and OmniScriptum S.R.L publishing group

120 High Road, East Finchley, London, N2 9ED, United Kingdom
Str. Armeneasca 28/1, office 1, Chisinau MD-2012, Republic of Moldova, Europe
Printed at: see last page
ISBN: 978-620-7-89933-3

I dedicate it to God, the source of all my wisdom, to my husband Giuliano Cordeiro for his encouragement and support, and to my sons Guilherme and Vinícius, inspirations for my professional growth.

SUMMARY

PRESENTATION

The global scenario shows a demographic profile with a large number of elderly people, which is a reality associated with numerous present and future challenges.

It is a privilege for me to comment on the relevant book by Kélvia Coelho Campos de Paula and Zélia Maria de Sousa Araújo Santos, which resulted from the dissertation *"Cnnuulta de enfermagem - tecnologia educativa em saúde para o autocuidado da pessoa com hipertensão arterial"*. Mainly because I know the trajectory of these nurses who have vast experience in providing comprehensive care for family members.

The authors recognise that the rapid scientific and technological advances of recent decades have contributed to radical changes in people's lifestyles and to the alteration of the population pyramid. There has been a progressive increase in the adult and elderly population, who have an increased risk of developing chronic diseases, which often have preventable or treatable causes, but high mortality rates.

The authors' experience has made them sensitive to the comprehensiveness of care for people with Systemic Arterial Hypertension (SAH), users of primary care services. This sensitivity allowed them, on the one hand, to realise that nursing care for this user needs to take into account that self-care is often related to self-perception and family perception of the disease and the meaning attributed by each of them to the experience of SAH, among other factors. On the other hand, their professional experience highlighted to them the urgency of the nurse's role in the nursing consultation being focused on a systematised and comprehensive practice centred on enhancing knowledge and skills related to promoting self-care for people with SAH, based on the assumptions of Dorothea E. Orem's theory and on the Classification of Health System. Orem's theory and the Nursing Classification System: NANDA, NIC and NOC.

In this context, the authors developed an investigation centred on the Nursing Consultation as an educational technology that facilitates the identification of the user's care needs, the establishment of goals and strategies for the promotion of self-care and the maintenance of health. The research journey was arduous, mixed with contradictory feelings in the face of every difficulty or resistance, but the perseverance and ethical-professional sense of the authors in contributing to the quality of care made them achieve the goal that culminates in the publication of the dissertation.

We invite readers of this book to expand this Change into other areas of care, where systematic, scientifically structured practice with a single language can improve communication between nurses and other health professionals, increase the promotion, protection and maintenance of life, favouring the self-care of users, families and communities.

It is hoped that reading this book will instigate new research in nursing, especially for professionals who want to implement change based on scientific evidence and those who want to have a Practice Based on Comprehensive Care, using the Nursing Consultation as a strategy for building new knowledge, in the connection, co-participation and co-responsibility of the triad: user, family and professionals.

Prof Drª Henriqueta Ilda Verganista Martins Fernandes
Nurse. Specialist in Child and Paediatric Health Nursing, Master in Nursing Sciences. PhD in Education. Coordinator of the Mobility and Institutional Exchange Support Office. Effective member of the General Council of the Nursing School of Porto. Member of the ESEP Research Unit (UNIESEP) and the Health Technologies and Services Research Centre (CENTESIS). Lecturer on the Nursing Course at the Escola Superior de Enfermagem-ESEP, in Porto-PT.

CHAPTER 1

INTRODUCTION

Nursing Consultation (NC) is a private activity for nurses (COFEN, 2017) and is significant in the composition of health activities, and should be an integral part of the actions produced by the health service provision system. Nurses must deepen their knowledge and practice in the proposed methodology, with an emphasis on the specific clinical field of their area of expertise, while also developing educational and psychotherapeutic skills, because according to Santos; Silva (2002), CE should be a favourable space for the person's complaints to be aired, for the demands or needs for self-care to be identified in terms of the biopsychic and socio-spiritual aspects and the person's abilities to carry out these activities. It also involves an educational moment, which aims to prepare both the individual and the family for self-care, contributing to the promotion, protection, recovery and rehabilitation of health.

According to Resolution 0544/2017 of the Federal Nursing Council (COFEN), EC must be developed in nursing care at all levels of health care, whether in a public or private institution, considering that it uses components of the scientific method to identify health/disease situations, prescribe and implement nursing measures that contribute to the promotion, prevention, protection of health, recovery and rehabilitation of the individual, family and community, and is based on the principles of universality, equity, resoluteness and integrality of health actions (COFEN, 2017).

The Nursing Process (NP), NC or Systematisation of Nursing Care (SNC), synonymous terms, is organised into five interrelated, interdependent and recurring stages: Data Collection; Nursing Diagnosis (ND); Planning, Implementation and Evaluation. The NC must be based on a theoretical framework that guides data collection, the establishment of NDs, the planning of nursing actions or interventions and provides the basis for evaluating the nursing results achieved (COFEN, 2009).

According to Garcia (2016), the SC is an example of systematising care and should be the foundation, the founding and structuring axis of the construction of knowledge and, consequently, of professional practice (teaching, care, research and management), given that care is the object of study and work of nursing. Dantas et al. (2016) add that CE contributes positively to the growth of nurses' professional training, as a whole or individually, broadening their view of the health-disease process and enabling them to improve the quality of care provided to hypertensive patients.

Costa et al. (2014) state that nurses are fundamental in the Basic Health Unit (BHU), as they take on the role of guiding and directing in CE, since, by carrying out a comprehensive assessment of the individual, adult or child, they reinforce disease prevention and health promotion, as well as allowing those involved in care to take responsibility, based on the guidelines transmitted by the professional, which makes it relevant to think about the nurse's role in the development of health education actions.

The rates of knowledge about SAH in the population vary from 22.0% to 77.0%, of treatment from 11.4% to 77.5%, and of control from 10.1% to 35.5%. Given this fact, it is necessary to understand EC as a complex technology, centred on human care and the decision-making process, insofar as it demands knowledge and practice in human care (SILVA; FERREIRA, 2014).

Therefore, EC has become a necessary form of assistance, inserted in the context of Primary Health Care (PHC), regulated, which allows for the systematic and continuous monitoring of the user, favouring the bond with the community, multiprofessional work and the interpersonal relationship between the professional and the client and their family, but it still doesn't have much applicability (CAVALCANTI; CORREIA; QUELUCI, 2009).

One of these challenges stems from the Brazilian health situation, which has been changing and is characterised by an accelerated demographic transition and is expressed by a situation of a triple burden of diseases, namely the unmet agenda of infectious diseases and deficiencies, the significant burden of external causes and the hegemonic presence of chronic conditions, This summarises a health situation that cannot be adequately addressed by a healthcare system that is still too fragmented, reactive, episodic and focused primarily on dealing with acute conditions and exacerbations of chronic conditions (BARBIANI, 2016).

According to Barbianiet et al (2016), the fact that the composition of the Family Health Strategy (ESF) is restricted and demand is growing can lead to professional actions being shifted to necessary but routine functions of a lower level of complexity than the nurse's potential competences.

From this perspective, nurses' work is seen as being tied to technical work and focused on direct curative care, with an overload of work, whereas what would be expected in the context of primary care is a work process oriented towards comprehensive care, which leads to some challenges arising from the inapplicability or ineffective applicability of EC (SANTANA et al, 2013).

Bento and Brofman (2009) add that EC brings benefits to the community and provides guidance for favourable measures aimed at appropriately addressing the specific needs of users, making its implementation in current health services of fundamental importance.

In this context, throughout my professional experience in caring for people with systemic arterial hypertension (SAH), I have observed a lack of systematisation in the nurses' work, i.e. they don't use EC. In other words, they don't use EC, which enables systematised and comprehensive care for people's health needs. This is because there is a lack or deficit in self-care actions among people with chronic illnesses, particularly SAH, which has been a major challenge for the health team.

SAH is a multifactorial clinical condition characterised by a sustained rise in blood pressure levels equal to or greater than 140 and/or 90 mmHg. It is often associated with metabolic disorders, functional and/or structural alterations of target organs, and is aggravated by the presence of other risk factors (RF), such as dyslipidaemia, abdominal obesity, glucose intolerance and diabetes mellitus (DM) (MALACHIAS et al, 2016).

In Brazil, SAH affects 32.5%, around 36 million adults, more than 60.0% of the elderly, contributing directly or indirectly to 50.0% of deaths from cardiovascular disease (CVD). Along with diabetes mellitus (DM), its complications, including heart and kidney disease, have a major impact on the loss of labour productivity and family income (MALACHIAS et al, 2016). Cerebrovascular accident (CVA) and acute myocardial infarction (AMI) are the two biggest causes of cardiovascular death in the world. In Brazil, CVD is the leading cause of death, accounting for 10.0% of all deaths; AMI is the second leading cause of death, estimated at 8.4% of all deaths. In 2005, expenditure on CVD in Brazil was three billion dollars, with 30.0% of these diseases being the reason for hospitalisations in the Unified Health System (SUS), at an estimated cost of approximately R$165,461,644.33 to the public purse (BRANDÃO et al, 2012). The main risk pathologies are SAH and DM, which affect around 20.0% of the population over 70 years of age (MOURA; SILVA; CARNUT, 2011).

Nurses have been contributing to the production of technologies that enable an integrative, humanised and quality perspective, addressing the most prevalent chronic non-communicable diseases (NCDs) in order to provide basic care (ROLIM et al, 2015).At the same time, there have been changes in morbidity and mortality patterns, due to a decrease in general mortality and an increase in chronic degenerative diseases, including SAH, with increased vulnerabilities and greater possibilities of functional disabilities (SILVA et al, 2014).

It is necessary to work on the quality of care, organise health practices and provide access to services from the perspective of comprehensiveness, given the mortality coefficient attributed to CVDs, which was 129/100,000 inhabitants in 2011, considered to be the main cause of death in the municipality of Fortaleza (BRASIL, 2010).

In order to provide adequate care for people with hypertension, health services, especially Primary Care (PC), must establish different strategies. Among the factors in the organisation of services, free access must be guaranteed and the user must be given a comprehensive, continuous and responsible approach, establishing lines of care appropriate to each individual. The protocols set up in primary care must guarantee links to professionals and services, the individual's knowledge of the disease, its risk factors and the measures implemented to ensure adherence to the therapy instituted, including the adoption of healthy lifestyles, family and community support, in short, the empowerment of users (MALTA; SILVA, 2013).

Therefore, as professionals committed to care, it is necessary to build a relationship with the human being, using multiple technological options to help them engage in self-care.

So, given the problem of the individual's lack of self-care in relation to controlling hypertension and maintaining health in general, we decided to carry out this study with the aim of validating the Nursing Consultation as an educational technology for engaging people in self-care to control hypertension.

CHAPTER 2

OREM'S GENERAL THEORY OF NURSING - Theoretical and methodological framework

Theories in nursing are used to describe, explain, diagnose and prescribe measures for care practice, providing scientific support for nursing actions. For nursing to develop as a science and profession, theories, research and clinical practice must be linked. Furthermore, theories guide and assist nurses in identifying solutions to the problems presented by individuals. From this perspective, in order to verify the applicability of a theory in nursing practice, many models for analysing theories have been developed, which allow nurses to identify and critically select the best theory to use in different clinical and care contexts (LIMA et al, 2016).

Vitor et al. (2010) define theories as the result of the perception of reality, the interrelationship of its components, the formulation and intersection of the concepts of human beings, the environment, health and nursing care. Nursing theory is then defined as a conceptualisation of some aspect of nursing reality whose aim is to describe phenomena, explain the relationships between them and predict consequences or prescribe nursing care.

Orem's General Nursing Theory (1995) was based on the idea that individuals, when capable, should take care of themselves. When there is incapacity, the work of the nurse comes into play in the caring process.

The choice to adopt Orem's Theory (1995) to support the construction of the CE instrument aimed at people with hypertension was based on the understanding that these users go through profound changes in their lifestyle and emotional structure, expressed by physical, emotional and social maladjustments that can influence the adjustments needed to accept and live with the new health condition, making it necessary to implement strategies that favour and encourage the search for stimuli that promote self-care skills.

Orem (1995) started from a question that arose when she was working on a project to develop a curriculum for a practical nursing programme. She asked what conditions exist in the individual when someone determines that they should be subjected to nursing care. The answer obtained, when the concept was expanded to self-care nursing, brought the abstraction that nursing is an "other self", seen as an agent of therapeutic self-care, whenever that individual is not enough to provide the care they need (OREM, 1995).

From the author's perspective, health is considered a state of wholeness that encompasses the body, emotional reactions, mental development, attitudes and reasons, being a state of integrity and wholeness, constantly evaluated by individuals, who become responsible for their own well-being and for doing good for themselves and others. In this process, the individual recognises that self-care is one of the aspects of healthy living, as it involves carrying out actions directed at oneself or the environment, with the aim of regulating one's own functioning in accordance with one's interests, integrated functioning and well-being (OREM, 1995).

Orem subdivided her theory into: self-care theory, self-care deficit theory and nursing systems theory (OREM, 1995).

The Self-Care Theory describes self-care and emphasises that carrying it out helps to maintain the integrity of the structure and proper functioning of the organism, effectively contributing to its development.

In 1958, Orem described self-care as the performance or practice of activities that individuals carry out for their own benefit to maintain life, health and well-being. When self-care is effectively carried out, it helps to maintain structural integrity and human functioning, contributing to its development (ARAUJO et al, 2016).

In this context, the individual's competence for self-care and the capacity they have learnt (agency or power of action) are considered (OREM, 1995).

The Self-Care Theory presents three categories of self-care requirements or demands: Universal - care associated with life processes and maintaining the integrity of human structure and functioning; "Developmental" - related to human development processes and events occurring during the various stages of the life cycle; Health deviation - occurs in conditions of illness or injury (BARROSO et al, 2010).

Dorothea Orem describes the universal requirements of self-care, making an association with life processes and maintaining the integrity of human structure and functioning (ARAUJO et al, 2016).

The Self-Care Theory is based on voluntary actions that the individual is capable of carrying out, taking responsibility for looking after themselves for their health and self-esteem. Dorothea Orem defines self-care as the performance or practice of activities that individuals carry out for their own benefit to maintain life, health and well-being (OREM, 1995).

Embedded in this concept, self-care appears as the personal care required by individuals on a daily basis to regulate their own functioning and development. And it is precisely when some of the requirements for self-care are compromised that self-care deficits appear, as explained in the self-care deficit theory proposed by Dorothea Orem (1995).

The self-care deficit theory proposed by Dorothea Elizabeth Orem is applied to people with cardiovascular and chronic diseases, especially SAH and DM, in view of the possibility of them compromising the self-care capacity of the person affected (DOMINGOS et al., 2015).

The deficit of self-care can be interpreted as a relationship and not as a human disorder, but it is closely associated with the presence of human disorders, functional or structural, outlining the presence of nursing in care (OREM, 1995).

Since the concept of self-care deficit refers to the relationship between self-care and the need for self-care, it is contained in the Nursing Systems Theory, which, when recognised, activates a nursing system. Thus, for nursing to be legitimate, the self-care deficit must exist (OREM, 1995).

Orem, in his theory, establishes self-care by deviation of health, as an example, is requested in conditions of illness medical measures required to diagnose or correct the condition. This type of requirement is necessary when people are ill, with specific disabilities or incapacities (ARAUJO et al, 2016).

In general terms, the Nursing Systems Theory encompasses the Self-Care Deficit Theory and the latter, in turn, contains the Self-Care Theory. When a demand for nursing care is activated, a Nursing System is produced (OREM, 1995).

The main concepts of this construct are the theory's metaparadigms: Person/Human Being, a being that differs from other beings in its ability to communicate and act for its own benefit and that of others, to symbolise its experiences and reflect on its environment; Environment as the holder of the conditions that can affect, positively or negatively, the life, health and well-being of the individual, family and community, and is linked to the definition of Society, which is responsible, together with its members, for the individual's health (OREM, 1995).

For this reason, Orem (1995) defines the nursing system as the set of actions and interactions between nurses and users, categorised as totally compensatory, partially compensatory and educational support.

Fully compensatory - This is when the inability to self-care is attested and nursing is necessary, and they may be socially dependent on other individuals who are part of the group or family, enabling them to continue their existence and well-being (OREM, 1995).

Partially compensatory - In this case, the nurse and the client take on caring and other activities, with one or both of them participating in this process (OREM, 1995).

Educational Support System - The client takes on self-care activities, guided and monitored at all times. The nurse acts as a kind of consultant and educator (OREM, 1995).

Dorothea Orem's theory (1995) provides a comprehensive basis for nursing practice, useful in education, clinical practice, administration, research and nursing information systems. Its main concepts are: human beings, health, society and nursing. It defines when there is a need for nursing intervention, related to the affected conditions of the client or family member, in which the nurse acts partially or totally, but never ceasing to be the conductor, educator and guide of the care process.

Orem (1995) bases her theory on the promotion and maintenance of health, considering the holistic aspects of nursing care and the individual's responsibility in relation to the care process, making it a dynamic, versatile and effluent system in relation to its objectives, simple to understand but complex in its composition.

According to Orem (1995), all people are capable of acquiring knowledge and developing skills that make them active agents of their own care. Based on this premise, it is understood that monitoring hypertensive patients, carried out in such a way as to identify their deficits and care needs and provide appropriate guidance and information, will make it possible for them to maintain their autonomy.

Thus, the use of this theoretical framework is justified because it provides the theoretical foundations that make it possible to meet the perceived needs of hypertensive people, signalled by the universal, "developmental" and health deviation self-care requirements, the stages of which can be visualised in the SC.

CHAPTER 3

HEALTH TECHNOLOGY - A tool for social transformation

Historically, technology has been identified as knowledge that has been derived from techniques used by human beings to survive in the face of natural phenomena. Technology has both produced scientific theories that explain it and support pure science, as well as deriving from pure science that produces applicable knowledge, applied science, and from which techniques are developed to solve practical problems. It has become common to use the term technoscience, which expresses this intimate relationship between science and technology (LORENZETTI et al., 2012).

Technique, in the general sense of the term, comprises a set of rules appropriate to effectively direct a particular activity (LORENZETTI et al., 2012).

The history of technology dates back to around 2.5 million years ago, when people began chipping stone shavings to make claws, and the first elementary stone tools appeared, characterising what would have been scrapers and cutters made from chipped stone (KELLY, 2012).

The construction of railways and later cars and aeroplanes drastically reduced the distance; regions that were once remote suddenly became close, contributing to the import and export of goods. Spatial coordinates, what is meant by "far" and "near", took on new connotations, completely different from what they were for individuals in different historical periods (MARTINS; NASCIMENTO, 2016).

Another benefit provided by technology is electronic communication, which presents radical changes as a multicultural world gains ground on the monocultural world of yesteryear. Ordinary people are able to obtain information and get to know other countries and cultures through films, meeting immigrants or travelling (FEENBERG, 2015).

With the marked scientific and technological development following the Second World War, the health of individuals and populations came to be considered a right to be preserved, contributing to the economic complex and health systems expanding with the medicalisation of societies. The continuous growth in health spending, the production of new technologies and changes in the epidemiological profile of populations has led to the need to develop mechanisms for the production and incorporation of technologies into health systems (BRASIL, 2010).

The National Health Technology Management Policy (PNGTS) consists of a set of management activities related to processes of evaluation, incorporation, dissemination, management and withdrawal of technologies from the health system, with the responsibilities of the three levels of government and social control, as well as the principles of equity, universality and comprehensiveness, which underpin health care in Brazil (BRASIL, 2010).

Health Technology are medicines, materials, equipment and procedures, organisational, educational, information and support systems, programmes and care protocols, through which health care is provided to the population, according to Ordinance No. 2.510/GM of 19 December 2005 (BRASIL, 2010).

In other words, technologies can be characterised by tools, equipment, artefacts or technological devices built for a variety of tasks and which emerge in people's daily lives, causing new concepts to be incorporated and reflected in people's way of living, taking on a character of speed, agility and efficiency (SILVEIRA; VALMORBIDA, 2016).

Technological innovations have stood out in the process of transformations that have been taking place in the world of work since the 1970s in capitalist countries, and since the 1990s in Brazil, and have strongly influenced the health sector. This process has included new material technologies such as new work equipment and instruments, new materials, advances in genetics and human reproduction. The sector has also been sensitive to changes in the structure of healthcare institutions (from vertical organisations to network structures) and in the ways in which the workforce is hired, under the influence of outsourcing and contractual flexibilisation, generally leading to job insecurity (SILVEIRA; VALMORBIDA, 2016).

Although the health sector is sensitive to and influenced by current changes, the number of studies on the subject is still small, especially with regard to its effects on increasing or decreasing the workloads of professionals in the area (SILVEIRA; VALMORBIDA, 2016).

These aspects are major challenges for nurses trying to maintain a balance between the objective and subjective dimensions of nursing care mediated by technology. The objective dimension refers to the application of structured knowledge and concerns the manipulation of machines and the interpretation of information derived in such a way as to direct actions, while the subjective dimension gains strength from all the expressiveness of caring (SILVA; FERREIRA, 2014).

The majority of technological productions recorded in the health area are aimed at the practice of care, however, the incorporation of technology can lead to the depersonalisation of the client, with a reduction in interactions with the team during the care provided. In addition, disadvantages can arise, such as unforeseen adverse events caused by drug therapy, ethical problems, the need for constant training to make professionals capable of handling them and heavy financial investment (GOMES et al, 2017).

Nowadays, the influence of technological innovation, whether in terms of the availability of equipment or new care techniques, on different fields or specialities in the health sector is also notable. This has had an impact on clinical and epidemiological knowledge, mental health, the cultural dimension of the health-disease process and work organisation and management models (SALAZAR; PINZÓN; MARTÍNEZ, 2014).

The health sector, strongly influenced by the paradigm of positive science, has been sensitive to the incorporation of material technology for therapeutic, diagnostic and life-sustaining purposes, using IT knowledge and products, new equipment and materials, but has been less aggressive in the use of non-material innovations, especially innovations in the field of work organisation and relations (LORENZETTI et al., 2012).

Educational technology has stood out for providing education and health promotion to the CVD population by allowing the systematic identification of the development, organisation or use of educational resources and the handling of these processes, as well as the use of techniques guided by equipment or the aid of audiovisual resources in the educational setting (SOUZA; MOREIRA; BORGES, 2014).

Researchers base health technologies on soft technologies, which are relational, such as welcoming and sensitive listening; hard technologies, such as well-structured knowledge that operates in the health work process, such as clinical medicine and epidemiology; and hard technologies, such as equipment and organisational structures (ENGELA et a., 2018).

Technologies are linked to consumerism, sexuality, behaviour and lifestyle, child development, learning and the effects on mental health (SALAZAR; PINZÓN; MARTÍNEZ, 2014).

Technologies bring new products and services to human daily life, which go beyond social interaction, in terms of the application of sociability, leisure, family, emotional and social relationships, bringing quality of life in terms of the ability to learn and build new life projects and citizenship in terms of the user's technological and digital inclusion (CHERNICHARO, 2018).

Among the technologies, information technology is of fundamental importance and needs to be adapted to, with the individual having to adapt to the new processes of change, because feeling included, involved in the development of society in the current dynamic, connected to the modern world, directly influences people's health. Health here is understood in its broadest sense, of physical, mental and social well-being, of inclusion, as an organising concept of lifestyle and quality of life, of the social environment and of living fully. Therefore, if the individual is not fully integrated into society, taking advantage of the opportunities that the current reality gives them, this can generate a feeling of alienation, leading to discontent and unhappiness, which interferes with their health (FEENBERG, 2015).

When it comes to health care, we have to take responsibility for a large part of the quality of the assistance provided, putting all the technological options we have in terms of knowledge at the service of the user. We must use everything we have to defend life, as possessors of the best that health technology has to offer, which is our knowledge, using multiple technological options to tackle different health problems. In this way, we emphasise nursing knowledge as technology, with the act of caring being the soul of health services, since the object of health is not protection and promotion, but the production of care, through which it is possible to achieve healing and well-being (FEENBERG, 2015).

Technological strategies should be used that range from individualised care to collective care with groups of users. However, despite the fact that technology is increasingly becoming part of the way people relate to each other and to the environment, the inclusion of technology in healthcare practice must be adapted to meet the social demands of contemporary life and reflect on the ethical issues that permeate the use of technologies in the face of intersubjectivity in the moment of care that goes beyond the technological (FEENBERG, 2015).

CHAPTER 4

NURSING CONSULTATION - Educational technology for self-care

Nurses use clinical judgement and scientific knowledge through the Nursing Consultation (CE), based on Law no. 7.498/86, established by Annex I of Ordinance no. 648/2006, later amended by Ordinance no. 1.625/2007 of the Ministry of Health and, since 1993, based on the Resolution of the Federal Nursing Council (COFEN), CE has become mandatory at all levels of health care in public and private institutions (ALENCAR et al, 2017).

EC has been implemented with the aim of uniting nursing activities, so that they are no longer isolated actions and become part of a process. Its use as a scientific working method makes it possible to improve the quality of nursing care through individualised action planning, enabling continuity and comprehensive care (SCHMITZ et al, 2016).

The EC enables nurses to assess the client's needs, as well as the variables that interfere with their treatment, allowing a space for discovery and interaction, favouring a more precise approach that is closer to the user's reality. However, the quality of this consultation can be influenced by factors that include the professionals' personal difficulties, as well as the health institution's structural and organisational ones (ALENCAR et a., 2017).

CE guided by self-care orients care practice through three pillars: adequate clinical management of the chronic disease; necessary changes in lifestyle; and valuing the client's emotional aspects, including changes in their vision of the future, or the way they deal with and cope with the chronic condition and its adversities (TESTON et al, 2017).

In order to recognise nursing as a science, it is essential to use NC, considering the essence of nursing. It is the dynamic of systematised and interrelated actions aimed at assisting human beings, characterised by the articulation and dynamism of its phases: nursing history, nursing diagnosis, care plan, nursing prescription, evolution and prognosis (DANTAS; SANTOS; TOURINHO, 2016).

CE presents the scientificity of the work of this profession, as well as supporting decision-making, predicting and evaluating the consequences of its application by nurses in the health-disease process of the individual, family and community (DANTAS; SANTOS; TOURINHO, 2016).

CE is a care methodology that provides nurses with tools to apply technical, scientific and human knowledge to care at the various levels of healthcare (XAVIER et al, 2018).

Xavier et al (2018) state that EC is extremely important, as it enables adequate care for users, which is necessary to obtain a unique therapeutic plan. In addition, knowledge on this subject is favourable for directing the activities to be carried out by nurses and their teams, according to the health needs identified based on the health problems of each client.

Systematisation has a direct impact on professional autonomy when it comes to care, and is standardised and accepted as a universal nursing practice. Nursing gains immeasurably from the application of NC, as it allows for the assessment of human needs in relation to biological, psychological, social, family and collective needs, enabling professionals to use their autonomy and participate in a problem-solving manner in healthcare practices (PINTO; RODRIGUES, 2018).

The nurse is emphasised as having all the necessary elements to care for others. Authors also state that any nursing action aimed at recovering the individual's full self-care can be traced back to the importance of the assumptions, methods and goals of the self-care deficit theory proposed by Orem (LOPES et al, 2015).

Schmitzet et al. (2016) show, in the literature and in everyday experiences of implementing SC in Nursing, the need for nurses to be based on theoretical support, in other words, to define a nursing theory that is consistent with the reality of the clients they serve in their organisational environment, in order to support SC, thus giving meaning to the universe of Nursing. This body of knowledge has been transformed, taking on different modes of expression in its construction trajectory.

CE is a methodological tool that guides professional nursing care and the documentation of the work process, organising professional work in terms of method, personnel and instruments, making it possible to operationalise it (DOTTO et al, 2017).

CE gives visibility to nursing's contribution to health care in any environment where professional practice takes place, whether in service-providing institutions, hospitalisation or outpatient services, schools, homes, among others (DOTTO et al, 2017).

It is therefore necessary to place greater value on primary care, abandoning the current medicocentric and hospitalocentric system, which causes overcrowding in urgent and emergency care units in municipalities where the primary healthcare network is not properly organised. The Family Health Programme (PSF) is a way of bringing more effective care to the population, without them having to go to a health centre (PEREIRA; FERREIRA, 2014).

In short, it is believed that the only way to increase people's confidence in EC is to use it more and more as a work strategy, including it in health programmes and valuing it as an instrument capable of providing increasingly effective, dignified and humanised care to the population as an instrument of self-care (PEREIRA; FERREIRA, 2014).

EC is a technology that works by improving self-care as it allows the individual to develop their own skills to improve their quality of life. It is the method in which the professional nurse has complete autonomy to develop comprehensive care strategies to promote the health of the client, family or community (DOTTO et al, 2017).

CHAPTER 5

SYSTEMIC ARTERIAL HYPERTENSION - A Public Health Problem

In Brazil, diseases of the circulatory system are the main cause of death, with a downward trend. Studies show that 7.6 million deaths worldwide were attributed to high blood pressure (BP), 54% of which were due to strokes and 47.0% to ischaemic heart disease (IHD) (MALTA et al, 2015).

SAH has a high prevalence and is considered one of the main modifiable risk factors for cardiovascular disease and one of the most important public health problems. Research has shown that the detection, treatment and control of hypertension are fundamental to reducing its effects; therefore, early diagnosis and maintaining adherence to treatment are cost-effective measures that benefit public health (MALTA et al, 2015).

SAH is a multifactorial clinical condition characterised by sustained high blood pressure levels >140 and/or 90 mmHg. It is often associated with metabolic disorders, functional and/or structural alterations of target organs, and is aggravated by the presence of other risk factors (RF) such as dyslipidaemia, abdominal obesity, glucose intolerance and diabetes mellitus (DM). It maintains an independent association with events such as sudden death, cerebrovascular accident (CVA), acute myocardial infarction (AMI), heart failure (HF), peripheral arterial disease (PAD) and chronic kidney disease (CKD), both fatal and non-fatal (SBC, 2016).

Despite the scientific consensus on the magnitude and impact of hypertension, which makes it a serious public health problem, control rates are still low. In Latin America and Africa, they range from 1.0% to 15.0%, while in Germany the SAH control rate among primary care users is 64.0% of all hypertensive patients and 18.5% among the elderly. In Italy, a longitudinal study reveals control rates of around 52.0%, while in Canada, which has the best indicator in the world, attributed to follow-up by primary care and an ongoing education programme for professionals, 66.0% have controlled hypertension (ZANGIROLANI et al, 2018).

CVDs are also responsible for a high frequency of hospitalisations, with high socio-economic costs. Data from the Hospital Information System (SIH) of the Unified Health System (SUS) show a significant reduction in the trend of hospitalisations for SAH, from 98.1/100,000 inhabitants in 2000 to 44.2/100,000 inhabitants in 2013 (SBC, 2016).

Weber et al. (2014) highlight the following as risk factors associated with SAH: age, in which there is a direct and linear association between ageing and the prevalence of SAH; gender and ethnicity, in which the prevalence of self-reported SAH was statistically different between the sexes, being higher among women (24.2%) and blacks (24.2%), compared to brown adults (20.0%), but not whites (22.1%); Overweight and obesity, salt and alcohol intake, a sedentary lifestyle, as well as economic and genetic factors also contributed to the rise in blood pressure levels.

Considering that the BP values obtained by different methods have different levels of abnormality, the abnormality values defined for each of them are used to establish the diagnosis. When office measurements are used, the diagnosis should always be validated by repeated measurements, under ideal conditions, on two or more occasions, and confirmed by measurements outside the office (ABPM), with the exception of those individuals who already have target organ damage (TOR) detected. Uncontrolled hypertension is defined when, even under antihypertensive treatment, the user's BP remains high both in and out of the clinic, as shown in the table below.

Chart 1 - BP classification according to casual or in-office measurement from the age of 18.

Classification	SBP (mm Hg)	DBP (mm Hg)
Normal	≤120	≤80
Pre-hypertension	121-139	81-89
Stage 1 hypertension	140-159	90-99
Stage 2 hypertension	160-179	100 - 109
Stage 3 hypertension	≥180	≥ 110

Note: When SBP and DBP are in different categories, the higher should be used to classify BP. **Isolated systolic hypertension is** considered **if SBP > 140 mm Hg and DBP < 90 mm Hg, and should be classified** into stages 1, 2 and 3 (SBC, 2016).
Source: (JAMES **et al.**, 2014).

Because it is chronic and silent, sufferers find it difficult to realise the problem, and this invisibility of SAH further compromises quality of life. In addition to the serious damage it causes to the human body, such as aggravating cerebrovascular disease, coronary artery disease, chronic heart and kidney failure and vascular disease of the extremities, it requires highly complex hospitalisations and technical procedures for its control and treatment, which has serious consequences for the individual, their family and society, such as absenteeism from work, deaths and early retirements (MARIOSA et al, 2018).

Given the impact caused by uncontrolled BP and the associated factors, it is worth highlighting the need for knowledge on the part of health services and professionals about individualised care for each subject, based on the general characteristics of this population group and knowledge about the classification of the disease (GOMES et al, 2018).

In this sense, the care provided to the individual, through routine consultations, allows the health professional to get to know concrete aspects of the user's life that directly influence

about pharmacological and non-pharmacological treatment, such as adverse effects of medication, lifestyle habits, degree of family support and blood pressure control. By valuing these aspects, professionals can identify the gaps between the education offered and the self-care carried out, reinforcing at each meeting, if necessary, the objectives and goals to be achieved in order to promote healthy lifestyle habits, which are essential for controlling the disease (BARRETO et al, 2018).

In this respect, difficult blood pressure control has raised the need for substantial strategies related to the care provided, coping and living with the disease. The diversity of factors that interfere with the treatment and control of hypertension, such as behavioural determinants, nutritional status, sociodemographics and adherence to pharmacological therapy, should be taken into account in the creation and adoption of new strategies, with periodic assessment of people by health professionals. In this sense, knowing the factors associated with inadequate BP can help to discuss and improve the organisation of the care work process, based on the population's health needs, with precise, effective and resolutive actions (RÊGO et al., 2018).

These findings reinforce the importance of the investments being made, not only in Brazil, but also around the world, to tackle Chronic Non-Communicable Diseases (CNCDs) such as SAH, beyond drug treatment, since there is scientific consensus about the positive effects of lifestyle changes and frequent monitoring of these. However, it is necessary to overcome the normative logic of the actions still dominant in the services, as pointed out by Gomes et al. (2018), in reference to educational approaches with SAH patients. This is because the qualification of services is linked to the efficiency of control.

The Ministry of Health (MoH) and the SBC suggest adopting actions that encourage the practice of self-care, with a cognitive and behavioural approach to the user, in order to assess their food consumption and in such a way that changes can occur without impacting on the social, economic, family and religious dynamics of these people (RÊGO et al, 2018).

The bond is the result of a process of interaction between the health professional and the user, which gradually consolidates and shares the responsibility of both in the health-disease process. In this process, the bond is a tool that strengthens the exchange of knowledge, scientific and popular knowledge, which together integrate the professional-user relationship and commit both parties to taking charge of healthcare. The bond becomes important for the qualification of professional practice in a broader perspective and in the control of chronic diseases, such as SAH, favouring self-care (KLAFKE; VAGHETTI; COSTA, 2017).

CHAPTER 6

METHODS OF CONSTRUCTION AND VALIDATION OF THE NURSING CONSULTATION - Educational technology for the self-care of people with hypertension

6.1 Type of study

This methodological study, according to Polit, Beck and Hungler (2011), refers to investigations into the methods of obtaining, organising and analysing data, dealing with the development, validation and evaluation of research instruments and techniques. The researcher's goal is to develop a reliable, accurate and usable instrument that can be used by other researchers, as well as evaluating its success in achieving the objective.

6.2 Place of study

The study was carried out in the 12 Primary Health Care Units (UAPS) distributed in the Regional Health Coordination II (SER II) in Fortaleza-CE. It should be noted that each UAPS had between 02 and 08 Family Health Teams (EqSF), as shown in Chart 2.

Chart 2 - Distribution of UAPS, according to number of EqSF, and Nurses in Regional Health Coordination II (CORES II). Fortaleza-CE, 2017.

UAPS	No. of FTEs	N^0 of Nurses
Aída Santos	03	03
Benedict Arthur	04	04
Célio Brasil	04	04
Flávio Marcílio	04	04
Friar Tito	04	04
Sister Hercília	08	08
Miriam Mota	03	03
Odorico de Morais	04	04
Paulo Marcelo	03	03
Pius XII	03	03
Sandra Nogueira	05	05
Rigoberto Romero	05	05
TOTAL	50	50

Source: Municipal Health Secretariat (SMS) - Fortaleza-CE, 2017.

In the state of Ceará, health care is organised into health macro-regions and micro-regions in order to comply with the doctrinal and organisational principles of the SUS (BRASIL, 2006; BRASIL, 2011a), which guides the process of decentralising health actions and services and the processes of negotiation and agreement between managers. The Fortaleza macro-region is the largest in the state. It covers approximately 70.6 per cent of the state's population, an estimated 6,032,600 inhabitants (SOUZA, 2013).

In the municipality of Fortaleza-CE, the Regional Secretariats (SR) are the sub-prefectures located in Fortaleza-CE. There are currently 6 (six) SERs - I, II, III, IV, V, VI. Each SER is subdivided into several PAs

(Private Areas), where superintendents, community leaders, secretaries and others work, with the task of guaranteeing a better life for the inhabitants and preserving the region's natural potential.

Fortaleza-CE has 109 UAPS, 402 Family Health Teams (EqSF), of which 2,458 are Community Health Agents (ACS); 341 nursing assistants; 389 nurses and 369 doctors. The Regional Coordination Offices (CORES) are made up of a superintendent who carries out the public policies defined by the municipal executive and provides services to the communities, being classified into I, II, III, IV, V and VI according to territorialisation.

It should be noted that each UAPS has a Coordinator. The number of Family Health Teams (EqSF) varies according to the number of families registered and living in the area, and each EqSF is made up of a nurse, a doctor, a nursing assistant or technician, and at least six CHAs, depending on the size of the assisted population.

CORES II is made up of 20 neighbourhoods: Aldeota, Cais do Porto, Cidade 2000, Cocó, De Lourdes, Dionísio Torres, Engenheiro Luciano Calvalcante, Patriolino Ribeiro, Joaquim Távora, Manuel Dias Branco, Meireles, Mucuripe, Papicu, Praia de Iracema, Praia do Futuro I and II, Salinas, São João do Tauape, Varjota, Vicente Pinzon, where 334,868 people live, corresponding to 13.50 per cent of the capital's population. This region of the city has an area of 44.42 km2.

6.3 Target population

Thirty (30) of the fifty (50) nurses who were members of the Family Health Teams (EqSF) allocated to CORES II in Fortaleza-CE and who monitored people with hypertension in the UAPS (Technical Judges) and ten (10) teaching nurses with masters or doctorates in the subject studied (Content Judges) took part in the study.

6.4 Validation of the Nursing Consultation - Health education technology for the self-care of people with systemic arterial hypertension

a) Presentation of the Nursing Consultation

The Nursing Consultation (NC) was based on the theoretical framework of Orem (1995). The NC contains five stages - data collection, diagnosis, planning, implementation and evolution/evaluation.

The following forms were used to carry out the CE: Data survey, which was drawn up by Santos and Silva (2002) and already validated; Nursing Care Plan (NCP), with the Nursing Diagnoses (ND) based on the Taxonomy of the North American Nursing Diagnosis Association (NANDA 20152017) listed according to Orem's "Self-Care Requirements" (1995) with the respective interventions and expected results, based on the NIC (Nursing Intevention Classification) and NOC (Nursing Outcomes Classification) (2012) as shown in Chart 3.

The EDs were selected a priori on the basis of the researcher's experiences of caring for people with SAH, and were the most frequently identified.

b) Validation of the EC

The EC was validated by two groups of participants:

1) Nurses who are members of the Family Health Teams (EqSF) (technical judges)

2) Committee made up of 10 (ten) content judges (JC) with extensive knowledge and experience in the subject and who are trained to analyse the content, clarity and understanding of the instrument (WOOD; HABER, 2014). The number of judges is in line with the recommendations of experts who suggest a minimum of five and a maximum of ten people (LYNN, 1986). The judges were selected based on the criteria for participation in the study. The search was carried out on the National Lattes Platform by refining the search with the criteria of master's degree or doctorate and area of work in SAH and educational technologies in health, in which the first ten CHWs who met the criteria were promptly selected and included. This was followed by the evaluation study in which the documents were distributed to the participants: Invitation letter (APPENDIX A); Informed Consent Form (ICF) (APPENDIX B) in two copies; CE - Data Survey (APPENDIX A); Instructional Guide for Nursing Consultation (APPENDIX B), PCE (APPENDIX C); Judges Identification Form (APPENDIX D), and CE Validation Questionnaire (APPENDIX E).

6.5 Data collection procedures

Data collection took place between January and March 2018, using the documents mentioned above.

To validate the content of this study, a measurement tool was used, the Likert Scale (1932), with five levels of support: 1-Totally agree; 2-Partially agree; 3-Indifferent; 4-Partially disagree; and 5-Totally disagree.

To collect data from the technical judges, a meeting was scheduled in agreement with the UAPS coordinator to explain the nature and purpose of the study, read the invitation letter (APPENDIX A), record their agreement in the Informed Consent Form (ICF) (APPENDIX B), followed by the delivery of the EC and the EC evaluation questionnaire (APPENDIX C). In the case of those who missed the meeting, the data was collected through visits to the UAPS where they were allocated.

For the collection with the content judges (JC), the Letter of Invitation was sent by e-mail (APPENDIX A). If they confirmed their participation in the survey, the ICF (APPENDIX B), the EC and the EC Evaluation Questionnaire (APPENDIX C) were sent via the communication vehicle of their choice (e-mail, conventional mail or in person).

The judges had up to 30 (thirty) days to return the data collection material. Those who didn't return the material within the pre-established period were contacted again, emphasising the importance of their participation, and given another 30 (thirty) days to return it. Thus, all those selected took part in the study.

6.6 Organising data

The data contained in the instruments answered by the judges was organised into themes: Characterisation of the judges, and Validation of the nursing consultation - Educational technology in health for the self-care of the person with arterial hypertension, and represented by percentages.

6.7 Analysing the data

The results were analysed based on the theoretical framework and selected literature. The judges' justifications complemented the analysis of the quantitative data and the suggestions that were deemed appropriate were incorporated into the Intervention Plan (IP).

6.8 Ethical and legal aspects

The research was carried out in accordance with Resolution 466/2012 of the National Research Ethics Commission (CONEP) (BRASIL, 2012), which regulates research with human beings. Participants were guaranteed anonymity and the right to withdraw their consent at any time. In order to preserve the anonymity of the participants, the technical judges were identified with the acronym JT followed by the numbering from 1 to 30, and the content judges with the acronym JC followed by the numbering from 1 to 10. The data was collected after the signing of the Free and Informed Consent Form (FICF) (APPENDIX B) and the issue of a favourable opinion from the Research Ethics Committee of the University of Fortaleza - UNIFOR, under number 2.542.700.

CHAPTER 7

RESULTS OF THE NURSING CONSULTATION VALIDATION PROCESS - Educational technology for the self-care of people with hypertension

To process the analysis, the results were divided into: Characterisation of the judges, and Validation of the "Nursing consultation - Educational health technology for the self-care of hypertensive users".

Characterisation of the judges

The majority of technical judges (TS) (96.67%) were female, had been working for between 9 and 13 years (90.0%) and specialised in Public Health (80.0%). All of them reported between 9 and 12 years' experience in caring for hypertensive patients. It should be noted that 26.6% of the JTs had a doctorate and 40.0% a master's degree.

With regard to the content judges (JC), 90.0 per cent were female, with between 9 and 14 years' professional experience (100 per cent), 50.0 per cent had a master's degree in Public Health and the rest had a doctorate in the same area.

Validation of the "Nursing consultation - Educational technology for the self-care of people with hypertension"

Feasibility/applicability of Nursing Consultation

Seventeen (56.6%) JTs totally agreed with the viability/applicability of the proposed Nursing Consultation (NC), justifying comprehensive care for the user, defining the nurse's role in relation to the object of work, and guiding the user towards self-care.

[...] excellent, long, but covers all aspects related to the patient and the pathology [...] (JT01)
[...] I think it's important for monitoring and treating patients [...] (JT 02)
[...] it's feasible, it allows us to get to know the patient's condition in a very comprehensive way [...] (JT03)
[...] very good as a form of primary prevention for secondary problems that may arise, very viable [...] (JT30)

Comprehensive user care is the result of a negotiation between managers aimed at integrating the various areas and actions in the programming of Health Care and Surveillance, seeking interrelated activities aimed at the specificity of the object of work with the identification of the main health problems, adding them to the strategies and actions of fundamental care for the diagnosis and monitoring of health problems (BRASIL, 2006).It makes it possible to integrate surveillance and care actions for SAH, taking into account programming, target control and monitoring.

Comprehensiveness is defined as a principle of the SUS which, considering the biological, cultural and social dimensions of the user, guides health policies and actions capable of meeting the demands and needs of access to the service network (BRASIL, 2006).

In primary care (PC), comprehensiveness is constituted in everyday work through the interactions that take place between users and professionals. So, considering comprehensiveness as one of the pillars of the SUS and taking the nursing workforce as an important contingent of people to operate in the construction of the SUS, it becomes important to identify what are the conceptual and practical bases that direct the work of nurses towards the construction of comprehensiveness in health (BRASIL, 2006).

Comprehensiveness emerges as a principle of continuous organisation of the work process in health services, which is characterised by the quest to broaden the possibilities of understanding the health needs of a population group. This expansion cannot be achieved without assuming a perspective of dialogue between different subjects and their different ways of perceiving the needs of health services (SILVA; BAITELO; FRACOLLI, 2015).

The instrument proposed by CE covers all the conceptual, practical and self-care requirements, because in our day-to-day work in primary care we carry out a merely practical or basic consultation with the hypertensive user, without following standards or aspects relevant to the EP.

> [...] it's excellent, I think we nurses should take ownership of what is rightfully ours and put it into practice [...] (JT12)

Pereira and Ferreira (2014) state that EC aims to provide systematised nursing care, identifying health-disease problems, carrying out and evaluating care that contributes to the promotion, protection, recovery and rehabilitation of health, from the nursing history to the physical examination, nursing diagnosis, therapeutic plan or nursing prescription and evaluation of the consultation.

According to Law No. 7,498/86, which states that EC is a private act of the nurse, capable of responding to the complexities of the individual, based on an accumulated knowledge of disciplines that also unravel human relationships (COFEN, 2017). According to the Federal Nursing Council's Resolution 159/1993, CE must be developed at all levels of health care, in both public and private institutions. This also includes the ESF, whose rules provide for the nursing interview (COFEN, 2017).

Implementing EC requires changes in nurses' care practices, so that they understand its complexity and realise that EC needs its own methodology and defined objectives. This change must come from the nursing professionals themselves, taking ownership of what is rightfully theirs, and not being at the mercy of an imposition tied to the "Reception Policy" to the detriment of programmes, prioritising acute events, transforming our Family Health Strategy (ESF) into veritable Emergency Care Units (UPA), which are not primarily aimed at promoting and preventing the population's health, but rather at immediate and brief rehabilitation.

> [...] applicable, as it guides nurses to engage in self-care for hypertensive patients [...] (JT 27)
> [...] it is important because it serves as a guide for the nurse and as a goal for the patient in their self-care [...] (E28)

[...] complex, applicable, complete technology, important for the self-care of hypertensive patients [...] (JT 18)

CE is a guiding principle for leading users to engage in self-care, which encourages people to adopt behaviours that are favourable to their quality of life, as nurses and the population share knowledge, promoting reflection on their actions and lifestyle habits.

The user becomes responsible for their own care, and health education is the main tool for building a working practice that values the human being beyond the biological, giving value to the social, emotional and spiritual being, given that health education involves the educational aspect.

However, 13 (43.4%) JTs partially agreed with the feasibility/applicability of the EC on the agenda, due to the prioritisation of prompt care (reception) in the UAPS, and the reduced time for the EC.

> [...] given the current scenario, where there is a prioritisation of emergency care (reception) in the UAPS, with a reduction in the workload allocated to scheduled demand (programmes), this instrument will have its applicability reduced [...] (JT 6)

> [...] very good and relevant, but extensive, due to the system imposed by the government which prioritises acute events rather than scheduled demands (JT 9)

> [...] in the system currently imposed in the UAPS, in which acute events are prioritised to the detriment of Ministry of Health programmes, this technology will be of little use (JT 14).

PHC is the set of individual, family and collective health actions that involve promotion, prevention, protection, diagnosis, treatment, rehabilitation, harm reduction, palliative care and health surveillance, developed through integrated care practices and qualified management, carried out with a multi-professional team and aimed at the population in a defined territory, over which the teams assume health responsibility (BRASIL, 2017).

Family Health is the priority strategy for expanding and consolidating PC, but it recognises other strategies for organising PC in the territories, which must follow the principles and guidelines of the SUS, configuring a progressive and unique process that considers and includes local and regional specificities, highlighting the dynamism of the territory and the existence of specific, itinerant and dispersed populations, which are also the responsibility of the team while they are in the territory, in line with the policy of promoting equity in health (BRASIL, 2017).

PHC considers the person in their singularity and sociocultural insertion, seeking to produce comprehensive care, incorporate health surveillance actions, which is a continuous and systematic process of collecting, consolidating, analysing and disseminating data on health-related events, and aims to plan and implement public actions for the protection of the population's health, the prevention and control of risks, injuries and diseases, as well as health promotion (BRASIL, 2017).

It will be up to each municipal manager to analyse the demand in the territory and what the UAPS offer in order to measure their capacity to provide solutions, adopting the necessary measures to increase access, quality and the ability of the teams and their services to provide solutions.

However, given the current scenario, there is a need to reorganise the current care model for monitoring hypertensive patients, focusing on ministerial programmes, seeking to reorganise the work process of the EqSF in order to improve the care provided, guaranteeing full, equal and universal access to healthcare.

> [...] not very feasible, as we currently only have 15 minutes to attend to each hypertensive patient [...] (JT 08)
>
> [...] given the current model in which we work with 15-minute appointments, it's not very viable [...] (JT 21)
>
> [...] it's feasible, as long as the consultation has an extensive timetable appropriate to its complexity (JT 05)

CE is an important tool in the health-disease process, facilitating the identification and solution of problems, being an effective and individualised specific scientific method appropriate to the particular needs of each user, enabling the quality of care provided that demands time and scientific knowledge (DOTTO et al., 2017).

In the current model, ECs are scheduled to last between fifteen and twenty minutes, which is insufficient to systematise the bonding and health education actions that are important during the first and subsequent ECs.

UAPS managers and coordinators need to be made aware of the importance of EC for people, given its comprehensive nature, which could help reduce hospitalisations, medication costs, disability and early retirement. To this end, it is essential to manage the process of caring for and monitoring the demand of people with or without health problems.

For 8 (80.0%) JCs, the proposed EC should be incorporated into the electronic medical record, as it makes it possible to broaden the nurse's knowledge, it consists of a guiding principle for guiding the user towards self-care, it makes it possible to change the user's behaviour, and it favours meeting the user's needs.

> [...] I consider the implementation of the nursing consultation for hypertensive patients to be relevant and feasible. I suggest that this technology be included in the electronic medical records of primary care units, making it an obligatory part of hypertensive care [...] (JC01)

The Electronic Health Record in Primary Care (FASTMEDIC) was implemented as a tool to facilitate and contribute to the organisation of health professionals' work, provide more personalised care, guarantee online access to users' medical records during consultations, produce better distribution and use of consultations, enable the organisation of work processes in health units, helping to plan professionals' schedules, procedures and visits, and make it possible to control the prescription, dispensation and stock of medicines. The system also offers a care protocol for hypertension, diabetes, leprosy, women and children (FORTALEZA, 2017).

The system manages user access to the system, allowing control of which modules, programmes and system functions the user can access and according to their professional profile. Its use reduces the repetition of exam requests and referrals through parameterised validations and online access to the client's entire history during their visit. This translates into savings for the municipality. During the service, cases of users in need of preventive medicine and follow-up are identified (FORTALEZA, 2017).

FASTMEDIC uses digital odontogram technology for oral health care, allowing the care plan planned and carried out for each person to be recorded. It makes it possible to automatically issue the Outpatient

Production Bulletin (BPA) for billing outpatient procedures, based on the information contained in the system, as it is in line with the information standardised in the Ministry of Health's systems (FORTALEZA, 2017).

The electronic medical record (FASTMEDIC) is a very complex, easy-to-use, complete technology, with a range of options to be explored and which does not contain the EC as a compulsory screen.

> [...] technologies are very important tools for improving nurses' knowledge and adherence to self-care for hypertensive patients, so the research focused on nursing consultation is very complete and will help nurses in conducting the patient care process [...] (JC02)

CE makes it possible to broaden nurses' knowledge as it recovers their clinical practice, recognising life values, social conditions, ways of coping and solving problems, adopting attitudes that make it possible to know the individual's signs and symptoms in their entirety.

The complexity of the search for recognition of health needs generates comprehensive care, with a view to greater resolution of users' health problems, with the implementation of care centred on individual guidance, which makes it possible to add new knowledge for the facilitators, as well as making it possible to change behaviour by adopting a healthy lifestyle (MACIEL; ARAÚJO, 2003).

EC is an effective strategy for the early detection of health problems and the monitoring of measures put in place to ensure people's well-being. It facilitates the work of nurses during user care, making it easier to identify problems and make decisions.

> [...] facilitating the nurse's work process based on a specific care plan and according to the diagnosis evidenced for each patient, as well as encouraging them to carry out their own care according to their health needs [...] (JC04)

EC is a guiding principle for guiding users towards self-care, as it allows users to develop their own skills to improve their quality of life. It is a method in which the professional nurse has complete autonomy to develop comprehensive care strategies to promote the health of the client, family or community.

> [...] it is an excellent tool for self-care and converges with individualised treatment, which can lead to changes in the user's behaviour [...] (JC05)

It is necessary for nursing professionals to look for strategies that encourage hypertensive patients to change their behaviour, as the adoption of guidance measures alone is not enough to ensure adherence to hypertension treatment. The family should be approached about the need for information on the illness process in order to help hypertensive patients with their health-disease process, since chronic diseases bring limitations and changes in lifestyle that are difficult to adapt to, but which are perfectly compatible with maintaining the individual's quality of life (ARAÚJO; GARCIA, 2006).

The implementation of relational care technologies has proven to emphasise nurse/user/family interpersonal relationships as factors that lead to increased adherence to treatment, even when the resolution of structural service problems is unchanged, demonstrating the need for comprehensive, systematic and interactive care (ARAÚJO; GARCIA, 2006).

The individual has to be co-responsible for their care, and as the nurse agrees on a plan of goals for self-care, they will feel motivated and encouraged to follow it.

[...] care can be observed in obeying the steps of the nursing consultation for hypertensive patients with a focus on self-care technology with important requirements obeying the Nursing Process with a focus on the main needs of the patient aimed at results, as it involves joint efforts between patients and nursing staff, to obtain the desired results [...] (JC06)

EC favours meeting the user's needs with an emphasis on self-care with changes to lifestyle habits such as: diet, hydration, sleep/rest, physical activities, leisure, occupation, socio-spiritual life, etc. For Campedelli (2000), self-care is a holistic view of health and refers to the practice of activities carried out by individuals for their own benefit in order to maintain life, health and well-being. Self-care is directly related to the beliefs, habits, cultural practices and customs to which the individual belongs.

In order to achieve the expected goals/results, it is necessary to liaise with the health or multi-professional team (EqS) in order to carry out a broad, multifocal care practice that favours the satisfaction of the individual's needs.

However, 2 (20.0%) JCs partially agreed with the applicability of the EC, to the detriment of the time stipulated by management for user service.

[...] I think it's feasible as long as the consultation time is increased [...] (JC07)
[...] long instrument, very comprehensive technology in relation to the care of hypertensive patients, but not very viable for current care practice, because the consultation time is limited [...] (JC09)

According to the National Humanisation Policy (PNH), the inclusion of workers in management is fundamental so that they can reinvent their work processes on a daily basis and be active agents of change in the health service (BRASIL, 2013).

Nursing consultation - stages covered by Orem's "Self-Care Requirements" (1995)

Self-care is a set of activities that the user carries out for their own benefit to maintain life, health and well-being in a conscious and deliberate way (OREM, 1995). The act of caring is at the heart of health services, because the object of health is not to cure, or to promote and protect health, but to produce care, through which it is believed that it is possible to achieve healing and health, looking for the basic conditioning factors which are: age, gender, state of development, state of health, standards of living, among others (TRENTINI; GONÇALVES, 2000).

Self-care requirements are actions aimed at providing self-care and are important for maintaining the functioning and maintenance of the human body, such as: Universal, "Developmental" and Health Deviation. Universal Requirements refer to the phases of the life cycle of all human beings and must be interconnected, important for maintaining proper human functioning associated with factors such as food, activity and rest, elimination and excretion processes, human life and well-being; "Developmental" Requirements relate to human development processes that may influence the phases of the human development cycle such as: prematurity, birth, childhood, adolescence, etc.; and Health Deviation Requirements are those that may arise through illness or disability (OREM, 1995 apud SANTOS; SILVA, 2002).

In this study, the stages of the NC are contemplated in: Data collection - interview and physical examination; and Nursing Care Plan (NCP) - nursing diagnoses (ND), interventions and expected outcomes.

Data collection - interview and physical examination

The Data Survey was authored and validated by Santos and Silva (2002), referenced by Orem's Theory (1995).

This stage consists of collecting information about the health of the individual, family and community in order to identify the needs, problems, concerns and human relationships that are essential for drawing up a health profile with accurate and reliable information (TANNURE; PINHEIRO, 2011).

Data collection corresponds to the first stage of the NP and must be duly recorded in the medical record to provide the EqS with information on the user's progress, facilitating communication, documenting and testifying to the nursing actions carried out in legal proceedings and providing support for diagnostic and therapeutic behaviour. It also makes it possible to evaluate the nursing care provided and serves as a source of reference for students and professionals to learn from (CARVALHO et al, 2008).

The JTs (100.0%) totally agreed with the structure of this stage, highlighting the complexity of the information that enables the identification of the user's care needs in the various dimensions - biological, psychological and social, the scheduling of actions to maintain health and well-being, favours the establishment of goals and strategies for care, and in short enables quality nursing care.

> [...] it does, because it's a very comprehensive data survey. I didn't find any requirements that I needed to add [...] (JT 05)

> [...] it is well detailed, allowing the determination of whether or not nursing care is needed, and the establishment of which system will be used [...] (JT 06)

> [...] contains important stages for physiological and psychological assessment, adaptation and orientation [...] (JT 10)

> [...] important interconnected factors for the maintenance of life and physical, mental and social well-being [...] (JT 19)

> [...] technology proposed to all stages of the life cycle and life processes important for the maintenance and functioning of the human body [...] (JT 20)

> [...] it benefits us nurses so that we can set goals and strategies, because the technology covers all aspects of Orem - universal, developmental and health deviations [...] (JT 12)

> [...] important for quality nursing care, with effective results and greater awareness among patients and carers [...] (JT 23)

Data collection is subjective and objective, deliberate and systematised, with the aim of outlining the health status of the client, family and community. It is an ongoing process that starts from the first meeting with the user, and is a key element in identifying the needs, responses and individual problems of each human being (CARVALHO et al, 2008).

The aim of data collection is to find out about the nursing problems experienced by individuals, so that care is aimed at meeting their needs as a whole, and that care takes into account their individuality, with their specific beliefs and values (CARVALHO et al, 2008).

The JCs (100.0%) totally agreed with the structure of this stage.

[...] the data survey is very complete, taking into account all the requirements proposed in Orem's Self-Care, covering all aspects of hypertensive users [...] (JC03)

[...] the survey lists self-care in detail, its deficits and what nursing care would be needed to compensate for these deficiencies [...] (JC05)

[...] the data survey presented contemplates the assumptions defended by Orem in her theory, where she emphasises that self-care depends on essential factors and can be affected by basic conditioning factors. These requirements are related to the daily activities of individuals, which range from organic and vital factors, from maintaining a state of health to social interaction factors. I noticed the presence of these factors in the data survey [...] (JC09)

Nursing Care Plan

The Nursing Care Plan refers to the phase of SC in which the nurse identifies the interventions necessary for the user to achieve the expected results, based on the formulation of the NDs.

Nurses adopt a decision-making process from the ED to design interventions in order to achieve the expected outcome. Such linkages are important for continually evaluating and adjusting diagnoses, outcomes and interventions to match the unique needs of each person or population. To this end, the use of nursing taxonomies such as NANDA and their respective links such as NIC (Interventions) and NOC (Expected Outcomes) facilitate nursing judgements for care planning, based on knowledge and understanding of the data, obtained by assessing each user during data collection (CHIANCA, 2002).

Nursing Diagnoses (ND)

ED is a clinical judgement about a human response to certain health conditions and life processes, or a vulnerability to such a response, of an individual, a family, a group or a community (NANDA, 2015).

The ED is made up of two parts: a descriptor or modifier; and a diagnostic focus. Each diagnosis should contain a title and a clear definition; if it is only the title, it is insufficient, because it is important for nurses to know the definitions of commonly used EDs (NANDA, 2015).

The NANDA Taxonomy of Nursing Diagnoses provides a way of classifying and categorising areas of concern to nursing, i.e. diagnostic foci, in which 234 NDs predominate, grouped into 13 (thirteen) domains that include nutrition, elimination/exchange, activity/rest and coping/tolerance to stress (BELLINGER, 2014).

The JTs (100.0%) totally agreed with the selection of EDs, emphasising their importance in assessing the person's capacity for self-care in order to make them an agent of self-care, and in the establishment of strategies by nurses to provide self-care.

[...] based on the diagnoses, the nurse detects the activities in which the patients have greater or lesser difficulty, assessing the degree of dependence of the patient for care [...] (JT 03)

[...] makes the patient responsible for their own care, guides them on how to proceed in order to be independent whenever possible [...] (JT 04)

[...] proper diagnosis redirects treatment and self-care [...] (JT 10)

[...] the diagnoses identified make it possible to develop their own behavioural strategies [...] (JT 12)

[...] relate appropriate adaptations to changes in the patient's life cycle [...] (JT 18)

The ND is a process of interpreting and grouping the data collected in the first stage, which culminates in a decision on the nursing diagnoses that most accurately represent the responses of the person, family or human community at a given moment in the health and disease process; and which form the basis for the selection of actions or interventions with which to achieve the expected results (COFEN, 2017).

With regard to EDs, the JCs (100.0%) totally agreed based on the frequency with which they are identified among users.

[...] they are pertinent diagnoses and are widely used during the process of caring for patients with hypertension [...] (JC02)

[...] the nursing diagnoses listed for the nursing care plan provide the basis for selecting nursing interventions to achieve the results for which the nurse is responsible, based on the main health problems that the hypertensive patient may present [...] (JC06)

<u>Nursing Interventions</u>

Nursing intervention constitutes the nursing care actions needed to achieve good results. Nurses must focus their actions on the planning carried out, checking that each activity is necessary, constantly reviewing the prescriptions put into practice in relation to the responses and performance of individuals, in continuous and constant monitoring (SOUZA et al, 2016).

Twenty-four (80.0%) JT totally agreed with the Nursing Interventions as a result of the nurse's role in empowering the user for self-care, establishing a bond between nurse and user, and providing opportunities for teamwork in meeting the user's demands.

[...] efficiently prepared, seeking to reverse possible problems. I just believe that a specific service will be needed for this purpose, as it's a complex assessment for the time allocated to our consultations [...] (JT 01)

[...] they help the professional to see the importance of certain interventions because they intersect with various diagnoses [...] (JT 02)

[...] provides plausible and relevant guidance to hypertensive patients [...] (JT 08)

[...] it makes it possible to set appropriate goals for each patient [...] (JT 13)

[...] provides the patient with changes in eating habits, psychological, mental and social changes [...] (JT 27)

Souza et al (2016) emphasise that nursing staff need specific technical and psychomotor skills in order to be able to build a relationship of trust with people.

The goal of nursing is to care, to care for the human being as a whole, in their biopsychosocial and spiritual spheres of human behaviour, centred on biological needs that often go beyond these.

When prescribing nursing care, nurses must be aware of the importance of the related factors and defining characteristics identified when drawing up the ED, as they reverse the aetiological factors associated with the diagnoses and resolve the signs and symptoms, hence the importance of eliminating factors that will contribute to the appearance of human reactions that will be evidenced during the client's anamnesis and physical examination (DOCHTERMAN; BULECCHEK, 2014).

The Nursing Intervention Classification (NIC) is a clinical tool that standardises the language for documenting nursing interventions and helps professionals to select appropriate interventions. This taxonomy is ideal for nursing professionals (nurses, students, managers and teachers) looking to improve their knowledge and perfect their practice (JOHNSON, 2012).

Nursing interventions are a valuable technology that shows the foundation of nursing as a science, which should never be forgotten by professional nurses, as it makes it possible to show the importance of nursing in the care process, encompassing changes in the lives of those who undergo the intervention, generating consequences for the family (JOHNSON, 2012).

With the current changes in the current health model insufficient from the point of view of health care as a universal right and full exercise of citizenship, the concept of health restricted to the biological and individual dimension has proved insufficient to meet the demands proposed by the dynamism of the SUS, In 2009, the National Policy for Permanent Education in Health (PNEPS) was implemented to train and develop health professionals, with the aim of encouraging them to self-analyse and self-manage their work processes in accordance with the principles and guidelines of the SUS and comprehensive health care (BRASIL, 2009).

Nurses become permanent educators centred on tackling the problems that emerge in health services, making work, care, education and the quality of care essential and inseparable elements of their practice, as perspectives for questioning their actions, activating health teams' consistency plans and encouraging self-care. Therefore, it is up to the nurse educator-training and multiplier process to adapt the curricular bases to the new professional profile, and to adopt innovative didactic-pedagogical strategies that articulate the teaching-learning process of the student, focusing on comprehensive training and the principles of universal, comprehensive and equitable care, so that the student becomes more critically aware of their actions (BARRETO et al, 2018).

In establishing a bond between nurse and user, the JTs emphasised the active participation of the user in setting goals and making decisions.

> [...] strategic guide and orientation for the professional, patient and carer, evaluating goals [...] (JT 17)

> [...] because the interventions are compatible with the diagnoses and allow implementation by both (nurse and patient) [...] (JT 27)

> [...] provides self-care and a bond between the professional and the user [...] (JT 19)

> [...] a rich, enriching tool for nursing consultations with hypertensive patients [...] (JT 24)

The National Humanisation Policy (NHP) seeks to put the principles of the SUS into practice in the day-to-day running of health services, producing changes in management and care methods. The NHP encourages communication between managers, workers and users in order to build collective processes to confront relations of power, work and affection that often produce dehumanising attitudes and practices that inhibit the autonomy and co-responsibility of health professionals in their work and users in their self-care (BRASIL, 2013).

EC becomes a support as a bond of trust and respect is established in the nurse/user relationship, as communication is essential for better assistance to the client and family who are experiencing the care process, which can result in stress and suffering. To this end, nurses are trained to recognise the interaction between nurse, client and family, establishing attitudes of sensitivity and empathy between everyone, contributing to humanised care. In this context, nurses have a commitment and obligation to include families in health care. The significance that the family gives to the well-being and health of its members, as well as its influence on the disease, obliges nurses to consider family-centred care as an integral part of nursing practice (CARVALHO et al, 2008).

The nursing team must establish a relationship that goes beyond physical care, through humanised actions, favouring the client's recovery with quality. It is true that dialogue between health professionals, users and family members fosters a relationship of trust and good results for quality care. The person being cared for needs to know how to listen, be present and empathise with the other person. In this way, both are strengthened and can find a solution to the health problem. This leads to the humanisation of nursing care, with interaction between carers and family members (CARVALHO et al, 2008).

The JTs (100.0%) highlighted the opportunity for teamwork in meeting user demands, in liaising with other (EqS) professionals, which also results in the construction of new knowledge.

[...] technology that involves a multi-professional team in the self-care of hypertensive users (JT 14)

[...] a tool that can be used to build knowledge in each patient's reality (JT 20)

In healthcare, work is carried out most of the time by a team, in a form of collective work, with communication being essential to establishing interpersonal relationships and with a common denominator of teamwork, which stems from the reciprocal relationship between work and interaction. It is therefore essential that health professionals recognise the importance of dealing with interpersonal relationships, as these end up significantly interfering in the care provided to clients. Professional demotivation can negatively affect the provision of care, since humanisation and comprehensive care are based on listening to and understanding the individual being cared for (FERNANDES et al, 2015).

Teamwork doesn't always mean working harmoniously, but the difference lies in turning conflicts into growth, knowing how to work with differences in ideas or behaviour and therefore acting professionally in the presence of conflicts (BARRETO et al, 2018).

However, 6 (20.0%) JT partially agreed due to the lack of some professionals in the teams, limited time for CE, too many users to attend to and prioritisation of emergency care in the UAPS by central management.

[Unfortunately, some actions depend on the help of a multidisciplinary team. In my reality, most of the time this isn't possible, because there are incomplete Family Health Teams, and the NASF, which is sometimes incomplete, is also always overloaded [...] (JT03)

[...] it requires time and willingness on the part of local management to admit that there is very little time for consultation [...] (JT09)

[...] an essential instrument, but a long one, unfeasible for our reality today [...] (JT10)

[...] in the face of the reality in which we live in health units with an overwhelming workload, it is impossible to carry out a nursing intervention [...] (JT21)

It is therefore understood that promoting health is a cross-cutting strategy in which visibility is given to the factors that put the population's health at risk and to the differences between needs, territories and cultures present in our country, with a view to creating mechanisms that reduce situations of vulnerability, radically defend equity and incorporate social participation and control in the management of public policies (BRASIL, 2010).

However, over the years, the understanding of comprehensiveness has come to encompass other dimensions, increasing the health system's responsibility for the quality of attention and care. Comprehensiveness implies, in addition to the articulation and harmony between health production strategies, the expansion of listening by health workers and services in their relationship with users, whether individually and/or collectively, in order to shift attention from the strict perspective of their illness and symptoms to welcoming their history, their living conditions and their health needs, respecting and considering their specificities and their potential in the construction of projects and the organisation of health work (BRASIL, 2010).

According to the National Health Promotion Policy (PNPS), it is the responsibility of the municipal level to adopt the evaluation process as part of the planning and implementation of health promotion initiatives, guaranteeing appropriate technologies, enabling a line of funding for health promotion within the permanent education policy, as well as proposing a performance evaluation instrument at the municipal level, implementing appropriate structures for monitoring and evaluating health promotion initiatives, among other functions (BRASIL, 2010).

The JCs were unanimous in their total agreement with the pertinence of the interventions proposed for each ED, justifying their impact on achieving quality of life for users, maintaining health and meeting the user's needs in an individualised way.

[...] the interventions enable a better quality of life for the hypertensive user based on the nursing diagnoses identified because they contribute to the control of hypertension [...] (JC03)

The achievement of quality of life by users is the individual's ability to live fully, as Bullinger et al (2017) consider that the term quality of life is more general and includes a potentially wider range of conditions that can affect the individual's perception, feelings and behaviours related to their daily functioning, including, but not limited to, their health condition and medical interventions.

Maintaining good health requires the adoption of healthy behaviours, such as regular physical exercise, low salt and animal fat intake, vegetable consumption, abstaining from alcohol and tobacco, stress management and regular use of medication.

> [...] a correctly identified diagnosis allows intervention to be targeted, i.e. care becomes individualised, but according to the context and individual needs of that user [...] (JC07)

Attending to the user's needs must be individualised, because although the health-disease process is collective, its manifestations occur in individual bodies, just as there must be an apprehension of health needs. These are socially determined and constructed, but can only be understood in their individual dimension, expressing a dialectical relationship between the individual and society (CAMPOS; MISHIMA, 2005).

Although health needs begin with the individual, they may or may not identify them and express them to the health service, which in turn may or may not decode them as a demand to be met. However, the actions and practices of the services don't always meet users' demands. Listening to the needs of health service users allows professionals to expand their capacity to optimise interventions in relation to the problems brought by the population. To this end, it is necessary to consider that work processes should aim to meet the health needs of the social groups that make up a given territory (SANTOS, 2017).

It is also important for professionals to be clear about the concept of health needs, as this should be part of the universal contract for health workers. In this respect, it is believed that public health policies should be geared towards universal rights. Conceptualising, identifying and classifying health needs is of great importance to enable professionals working in the field of Collective Health to get closer to the phenomenon and plan their actions, with the aim of satisfying the population's health needs (SANTOS, 2017).

<u>Expected results</u>

Nursing assessment is a deliberate, systematic and continuous process of verifying changes in the responses of the person, family or human community at a given moment in the health-disease process, to determine whether nursing actions or interventions have achieved the expected result and to verify the need for changes or adaptations in the stages of the NP (COFEN, 2017).

Implementation is the fourth stage of the EC and means carrying out and investigating the user's own responses to their performance in carrying out the care imposed, requiring specific technical and psychomotor skills from the whole team, in order to develop a relationship of trust with the user (CRAVEN; HIRNLE, 2006).

Chianca (2002) states that the reliability of a diagnosis, a nursing prescription or an outcome should be based on the average level of agreement about the diagnosis, the outcomes to be achieved and the prescriptions for achieving the established objectives.

The Nursing Outcomes Classification (NOC) is a taxonomy that complements the NANDA and NIC taxonomies. It lists outcomes for each NANDA diagnosis (JOHNSON et al, 2012).

The NOC taxonomy determines the health condition of each user, carer, family or community, with the aim of verifying the changes they experience following nursing interventions (JOHNSON et al, 2012).

The results refer to a state, behaviour or perception of the individual, family or community that can be measured throughout the nursing interventions, according to the client's responses to the conduct carried out by the nurses, making it possible to identify improvements or worsening or even maintenance of the condition assessed, based on comparisons with the assessments carried out previously (JOHNSON et al, 2014).

The JTs (100.0%) totally agreed with the elaboration of the "Expected Results", with a view to adapting to the interventions listed, consequent to the EDs, and which make it possible to evaluate the user in relation to the effective practice of self-care actions.

> [...] they help the professional to see the importance of certain interventions, because they intersect in various diagnoses [...] (JT 02)

> [...] because they are also compatible with the diagnoses, they provide clarity as to the objectives that must be achieved [...] (JT 06)

> [...] if the nursing interventions are taken care of, the results will soon be achieved, and thus we can evaluate the patient's self-care, promoting their health [...] (JT 03)

Nurses are responsible for directing the service and management activities such as planning nursing care, consultancy, auditing, CE, prescribing nursing care, direct care for life-threatening clients, prescribing medication (established in health programmes and routine) and all care of greater technical complexity (COFEN, 2017).

According to the SUS Users' Rights Charter (2007), citizens are guaranteed the right to orderly and organised access to health systems, with a view to fairer and more effective care, adequate and effective treatment for their problems, with a view to improving the quality of the services provided, welcoming care and freedom from discrimination, with a view to equal treatment and a more personal and healthy relationship, care that respects the values and rights of the user, with a view to preserving their citizenship during treatment, the responsibilities that the citizen must also have so that their treatment takes place properly and the commitment of managers so that the above rights are fulfilled (BRASIL, 2013).

The JCs (100.0%) had the same opinion as the nurses with regard to the "Expected results", attributing them to congruence with the experience of monitoring the user, compatibility with SAH control and the possibility of user autonomy, coherence with the diagnoses that make health promotion possible, and the viability of the nurse's self-assessment with a view to their behaviour and the user's evolution through the practice of self-care actions.

> [...] the expected results, in my perception, are complete and very pertinent in the care of patients with hypertension, because they are what we experience on a daily basis, and they show results that we expect the patient to achieve after the interventions [...] (JC02)

The user must be responsible for ensuring that their treatment and recovery are adequate and without interruption, taking responsibility for providing appropriate information during appointments, consultations and hospitalisations about complaints, illnesses, medication histories, previous hospitalisations, state of health, expressing whether they have understood the information and guidance received and, if they still have doubts, asking for clarification, follow the treatment plan proposed by the professional or health team responsible for their care, which must be understood and accepted by the person who is also responsible for their treatment, inform the health professional or team responsible of any fact that occurs in relation to their health condition, take responsibility for refusing recommended procedures, tests or treatments and for failing to comply with the professional's or health team's guidelines (DOTTO et al, 2017).

> [...] Expected results are based on the goals proposed for the patient's own control, giving them the right to autonomy [...] (JC05)

The family is an important part of caring for individuals with chronic illnesses, as it can be considered a great ally for effective self-care, giving users the autonomy they need to improve their health-disease process (DOTTO et al, 2017).

> [...] based on the interventions identified in the nursing diagnoses, the expected results are coherent. I believe that when well orientated, the user will take the necessary actions to maintain their health and prevent complications from SAH [...] (JC06)

> [...] the *"Expected **Results**" allow the Nurse to evaluate the interventions and the evolution of the care provided by the users* [...] (JC10)

Consistency with diagnoses related to health promotion is based on actual or present problems, as well as potential or future problems, which can be symptoms of physiological, behavioural, psychosocial or spiritual dysfunction, being identified and listed based on the degree of threat and the user's level of well-being, thus providing a central focus for subsequent steps (CARPENITO, 2016).

The proposed educational technology (Nursing Consultation) enables nurses to lead people with hypertension to engage in self-care in order to control their blood pressure.

The JTs (100.0%) totally agreed with the EC proposed with a view to engaging users in self-care to control hypertension, highlighting the following relevant aspects: broad and comprehensive coverage, focusing on the individual; building new knowledge between nurses and users; and establishing bonds and co-participation between those responsible for engaging users in self-care - the users themselves, family members and professionals.

> [...] a *complete instrument that covers all the patient's environments, audiences, reactions, coexistence* [...] (JT 01)

> [...] *the technology (EC) shown makes use of various options for approaching the patient, facilitating their engagement in self-care* [...] (JT 02)

> [...] it *covers the patient in a holistic way, covering all areas - physical, social and emotional* [...] (JT 04)
> [...] *leads users to educate themselves about their own health, promoting complete physical, mental and social well-being, which defines health* [...] (JT 25)

Broad, comprehensive care focused on the person is a radical change in the healthcare model that involves not only prioritising primary care and moving away from the hospital-centric model and specialities, but above all focusing on the user-citizen as an integral being, abandoning the fragmentation of care that turns people into diseased organs, systems or pieces of people. Interactive practices must be available as care alternatives (SILVA; SENA, 2015).

Integrality means seeing the individual as a whole, as a biological, psychological, social and sometimes even spiritual being. Integrality is remembering that the individual is a complete being, an integral being, trying to look after the user as a whole, not just the part that is ill. Above the complaint, comprehensive care means looking at the illness as well as the social and psychological aspects; by talking, we can do this; assisting the client in every way: they don't just need a bandage, they need a chat, attention. Comprehensive care is health care as a whole, so that the person can live with their illness with dignity and be happy (CAMPOS; MISHIMA, 2005).

The World Health Organisation (WHO) defines health as "a state of complete physical, mental and social well-being and not merely the absence of disease or infirmity". Health has therefore become more of a community value than an individual one. Health services continually seek to broaden the possibilities of understanding the health needs of a population group, a broadening that cannot be done without assuming a perspective of dialogue between the different subjects and their different ways of perceiving the needs for health services (PINHEIRO, 2016).

The Self-Care Theory focuses on the importance of recognising the person as having the right to exercise control over themselves and their care. In self-care education, the individual must participate in the decision, taking into account their values, beliefs, level of knowledge, skills and motivation. When Orem defines the Nursing Systems for nurses to act on the basis of self-care deficits, the support-education system opens up the educational perspective for nursing actions (OREM, 1995).

Freire (2001) advocates an education in which people learn from their experiences, moving away from the traditional model of education in which they receive information from others who have the knowledge. Drawing inspiration from this author helps to develop a more humane, participatory nursing education practice that values dialogue.

> [...] an instrument that, if applied, allows for proximity and the construction of knowledge, making the patient understand and feel responsible for their care [...] (JT 06)

The construction of new knowledge between nurses and users takes place through educational support, based on participatory dialogue, in which everyone contributes to the formation of knowledge, learning and teaching. It's not just an educational moment, but also a time for establishing bonds of friendship and support, therapy and leisure. In this space, people can speak and be heard and understood. Educational practice is the construction of the care process, it is a contribution to the person with a chronic non-communicable disease, in the sense of making self-care a reality, which has repercussions for autonomy and well-being.

EC contains an educational care plan whose actions are classified as: doing, guiding, referring, helping and supervising, empowering both the nurse and the user in the system of caring, teaching and learning the health-disease process (PINHEIRO, 2016).

> [...] the patient and the professional start to have a greater bond, and the patient starts to take responsibility for their self-care in order to achieve their goals [...] (JT 14)

> [...] there is co-participation between the subject, the family and the professional. Everything favours the patient's involvement in caring for their health and illness [...] (JT 15)

The establishment of a bond and co-participation between those responsible for the user's engagement in self-care - the user themselves, family members and professionals - is characterised as co-management which, according to the PNH (BRASIL, 2013), refers to the inclusion of new subjects in the processes of analysis and decision-making regarding the expansion of management tasks - which also becomes a space for analysing contexts, politics in general and health in particular, as a place for formulating and agreeing on tasks and collective learning. The PNH highlights two groups of co-management devices: those that relate to the organisation of a collective management space that allows for agreement between the needs and interests of users, workers and managers; and those that refer to mechanisms that guarantee the active participation of users and their families in the day-to-day running of health units.

Increased commitment and co-responsibility between health workers, users and the territory in which they are located changes the way health services are cared for and managed, since the production of health becomes inseparable from the production of more active, critical, involved and supportive subjectivities and, at the same time, requires the mobilisation of political, human and financial resources that go beyond the health sphere (CHIANCA, 2002).

In this way, users educate themselves, adhere to and become co-participants in the treatment of their illness, which contributes to a good welcome that means recognising what the other person brings as a legitimate and unique health need. Welcoming must be part of and underpin the relationship between teams/services and users/populations (BRASIL, 2013).

According to the JCs (100.0%), CE makes it possible for users to engage in self-care because it establishes a therapeutic relationship between nurses and users and the latter's active participation in controlling their condition, it leads to health promotion, avoiding the need for specialist care, it encourages behavioural changes in users to control their hypertension and maintain their health, and it favours the user's commitment to their health.

> [...] the technology will provide integration between the professional and the hypertensive patient, as well as co-participation of the user as a protagonist in the control of hypertension [...] (JC01)

The establishment of a therapeutic relationship between nurse and user and the active participation of the latter in the control of their condition can help the individual to conceptualise their problems, face them, visualise their participation in the experience and alternative solutions, as well as finding new patterns of behaviour. The nurse-patient relationship, from a therapeutic perspective, is about: the individual's perception of the experience or situation (how the professional experiences her relationship with the client); the individual's perception of the other (how the nurse perceives the individual); and metaperception (what the nurse imagines or infers that the client is feeling or perceiving about her) (LAING et al, 2016).

> [...] the consultation provides comprehensive, theoretically-based guidelines (NANDA, NIC and NOC) that are adopted according to the PHC user's health needs, enabling them to engage in their own care, working effectively to promote health, preventing illnesses and instabilities, and avoiding, in most cases, unnecessary visits to secondary and tertiary care services in the care network [...] (JC04)

Health promotion is carried out, avoiding the need for specialised care, as interaction with the nurse makes it possible to interfere with their health problems and meet their needs. They also point to the need to place the client at the centre of the care process, including them in the gains and cures obtained through technical and scientific efficiency, with respect for their integrity and dignity, recognising them as a potential subject of interventions in the health context. Finally, they indicate that the way nurses experience their relationship with users influences their behaviour and actions in the workplace (BRASIL, 2010).

Silva and Sena (2015) cite three categories of health prevention/promotion as: Primary, when it is carried out by immunological factors, occupational health, personal and household hygiene, genetic counselling, vector control, accident prevention; Secondary, when already in the form of a disease, it is carried out on the individual themselves, including treatment, diagnosis with disability limitation; and Tertiary, aimed at preventing disabilities and rehabilitation.

> [...] in the consultation, there is the suggestion of behavioural change, eating habits, prevention and health promotion, etc. Despite educational barriers, access to the health system and other adverse factors [...] (JC05)

> [...] the technology proposal is comprehensive, aimed at hypertensive individuals, in order to help them become active subjects and carers of their health [...] (JC09)

The proposed technology (Nursing Consultation) enables nurses to lead people with hypertension to engage in self-care in order to maintain their health.

The JTs (100.0%) totally agreed with the EC proposed in engaging the user in self-care to maintain their health, since the orientated user will experience quality of life, the early identification of health problems will make it possible to prevent health risks, and the educational aspect makes the user an agent of self-care.

> [...] even if they need family support, the patient will have an easier quality of life with all the proposed guidelines [...] (JT 01)

> [...] it allows risk factors to be identified and nurses can act preventively [...] (E03)

> [...] once it leads the user to health education, they become agents of their own self-care, keeping them well informed [...] (JT 05)

The analysis of the health-disease process has shown that it is the result of the ways in which production, work and society are organised in a given historical context, and that the biomedical apparatus is unable to modify the broader conditioning factors and determinants of this process, operating a model of care marked, more often than not, by the centrality of symptoms (SILVA; SENA, 2015).

Maintaining their health works as a cross-cutting strategy that highlights factors that put the population's health at risk, with a view to mechanisms to reduce vulnerabilities in defence of equity, participation and social control in the management of public policies (BRASIL, 2013).

For Orem (1995), self-care is the practice of activities that the individual initiates and carries out for their own benefit, to maintain life, health and well-being. Its purpose is actions that, following a model, contribute in a specific way to human integrity, functions and development. These purposes are expressed through actions called self-care requirements. Therefore, the basic premise of Orem's self-care theory is the belief that human beings have their own abilities to promote self-care, and that they can benefit from the care of the nursing team when they are unable to self-care due to poor health.

Nursing care provided with a scientific basis provides subsidies and strategies for implementing actions that make it possible to improve the practice of caring for people.

In this context, educational practices should be carried out based on an educational model that provides an environment capable of stimulating the user's criticality and transformative capacity, in a way that understands all the subjects involved in the process as actors in the teaching-learning process, aiming to respond to all the demands pointed out by the subjective reality of each individual. Therefore, this approach focuses on the awareness and participation of the subjects, whose educators seek to evaluate and problematise their social reality (LAING et al, 2016).

The JCs (100.0%) totally agreed with the EC on the user's engagement in self-care to maintain their health, to the detriment of encouraging the search for knowledge and the adoption of healthy habits, the feasibility of the orientation and follow-up process, and the improvement of the nurse's performance in the user's health care.

> [...] technology will encourage and show that it is possible to maintain health through knowledge and healthy habits [...] (JC01)

> [...] hypertensive patients who are aware of their health problem end up adhering better to treatment, Technology contributes to this knowledge, so they tend to understand more about the disease, its risk factors and complications, as well as the importance of changing their lifestyle to maintain their health [...] (JC03)

The professionals seek to offer quality of life to people with SAH, encouraging them to be autonomous subjects of their actions, reflecting on their bodies based on knowledge about their health, with a view to modifying lifestyle habits in the quest to achieve healthy attitudes.

> [...] in the consultation, I believe that the professional will have the support to better accompany and guide the patient in the process of caring for their health [...] (JC02)

Feasibility in the process of orientating and monitoring users enables professionals to reflect critically and participatively on their work, significantly influencing their participation in the process of caring for individuals and their families.

> [...] the proposed technology will help to refine and improve clinical practice during nursing consultations so that nurses can guide users to engage in self-care in order to maintain their health and avoid complications in the future. It is suggested that a letter be drafted to municipal, state and federal managers, to be widely publicised in the Family Health Strategy [...] (JC06)

> [...] the tool addresses viable conditions for nurses to use in their routine care of hypertensive patients, favouring

the engagement of hypertensive service users to adopt measures that maintain and benefit their health [...] (JC09)

Improving nurse performance in user health care produces technological transformations that influence care, values, knowledge and skills, collaborating in professional improvement, influencing the client's life significantly in terms of engagement in self-care and health maintenance.

Contributions to the incorporation of the proposed technology (Nursing Consultation) into nurses' professional practice

The JTs (100.0%) reported the necessary conditions for incorporating EC into primary care: time to apply EC; availability in electronic format; periodic monitoring of EC application to assess effectiveness; space to record other EDs identified in the user; training for nurses to apply EC; publicising it in the Regional Health Coordinating Offices (CORES) of Fortaleza-CE; and making managers and administrators aware of the relevance of EC for users and nurses.

[...] I think it's important to emphasise the time taken to apply the instrument during consultations at the UAPS [...] (JT 01)

The time it takes to apply EC depends on each user, they are all individualised with unique pathologies, with different needs that often require more time to establish a nurse-client relationship, however, in the current health model imposed by the public administration, we work with diary systems with scheduled appointments lasting fifteen minutes for hypertensive/diabetic users, which is unfeasible for the application of EC technology, which requires a holistic approach to health and disease situations, as it seeks to prevent common problems such as nutritional disorders, respiratory and cardiovascular diseases, among others, through promotion and prevention actions (SOUZA et al., 2013).

[...] be done in virtual format, with multiple choices, because if it's normal it gets very tiring [...] (JT 02)

Making the EC available in digital format in the FASTMEDIC medical record would be ideal, as a compulsory screen for every consultation with hypertensive users, as a way of standardising and making consultations routine, redefining consultation times and reorganising the care provided to people.

With the digital format and the use of technology, it is possible to have access to a vast network of information in real time and also to exchange and cross-check data at any time. With the use of electronic medical records, services would be streamlined and facilitated, as the systems are interconnected throughout the capital of Fortaleza-CE, meaning that if a person is registered at a respective UBS, they will have access to other units with the same electronic record (FORTALEZA, 2017).

Any information can be obtained instantly, the visibility of facts has become greater and faster, where data is updated as a whole. Levy (2016) explains that the digital interface widens the field of the visible, highlighting the emerging evolution that has diversified, facilitated and transmitted information instantaneously and widely. The Internet has made citizens potentially interactors and communicators. Not only do they now have greater access to information, but they can also participate in it directly, giving their opinion and interacting at the same time as receiving it.

> [...] quarterly monitoring and group meetings to assess the effectiveness of the technology [...] (JT 04)

Periodic monitoring of the application of EC to assess efficacy is important for the ongoing process of analysing and summarising the health benefits, economic and social consequences of the use of technologies, considering the following aspects: safety, accuracy, efficacy, effectiveness, costs, cost-effectiveness and aspects of equity, ethical, cultural and environmental impacts involved in their use.

The decision to incorporate a new technology should take into account the comparison between the technology being analysed and those that have already been incorporated, in terms of the evidence of benefits, the costs to the system, the target population, the infrastructure needs in the health services network and the factors promoting equity (BRASIL, 2010).

> [...] propose new nursing diagnoses that will better contemplate the care provided to users in primary care [...] (JT 05)

The Ministry of Health is responsible for: coordinating the incorporation and exclusion of technologies within its sphere of activity; regulating the implementation of technologies in the healthcare network in order to guarantee access to all those who need it, under appropriate and safe conditions of use; supporting managers in the implementation of technologies; developing and improving systems that allow information to be obtained on the results and impacts of the use of technologies in healthcare systems (BRASIL, 2010).

Permanent education is education in which learning and teaching are incorporated into the daily life of organisations and work. Continuing education is based on meaningful learning and the possibility of transforming professional practices. Continuing education can be understood as work-based learning, i.e. it takes place in the daily lives of people and organisations. It is based on the problems faced in reality and takes into account the knowledge and experience that people already have. It proposes that health workers' education processes should be based on problematising the work process, and considers that workers' training and development needs should be guided by the health needs of people and populations. The aim of continuing health education processes is to transform professional practices and the organisation of work itself (BRASIL, 2009).

> [...] training of nurses before the consultation and demonstration of the proposed technology in regional health centres [...] (JT 29)

Training nurses to apply EC will involve the use of intentional and planned actions whose mission is to strengthen knowledge, skills, attitudes and practices that the dynamics of organisations do not offer by other means, at least on a sufficient scale, but training also develops under the influence of a wide variety of institutional, political, ideological and cultural conditions, which anticipate and determine the space within which training can operate its limits and possibilities (BRASIL, 2009).

Simplification, which reduces the problem of staff education to a question of applying pedagogical methods and techniques; the instrumental view of education, which thinks of educational processes only as a means of achieving a specific objective; immediacy, which believes in the possibility of great effects from an educational programme that can be applied quickly; low discrimination of problems to be overcome; the tendency to act through programmes and projects, whose logic is one of beginning and end, are examples of avoiding deviations within which training can operate with its limits and possibilities (BRASIL, 2009).

Nursing makes nurses feel fulfilled with the activities they carry out in the context of their work and in the eyes of society, developing their work with greater commitment and satisfaction, which motivates them to provide better quality care. Nurses become key players in planning, organising, executing and developing the teamwork process, which strengthens the process of recognising their identity and autonomy.

> [...] making managers aware of the need for nursing consultations for patients with chronic diseases, remembering that they require much more than a simple prescription renewal, but rather a detailed assessment [...] (JT 06)

Publicising it in the Regional Health Coordinating Offices (CORES) of Fortaleza-CE; and making managers and administrators aware of the relevance of CE for users and nurses as an excellent strategy for improving the health of users, families and the community. According to the National Health Technology Management Policy (PNGTS), technology is the ideal means of disseminating information through instruments that take into account the target audience and the appropriate language, the time available for evaluation, transparency and the explanation of conflicts of interest, as shown in the National Health Technology Management Policy (BRASIL, 2010).

According to the Municipal Guidelines for Hypertension Control (2014), attending hypertensive patients every three months generates serious cardiovascular and disability problems for this class, which could be solved by adopting a previous CE, with the commitment of professionals and managers to incorporate new strategies and care technologies aimed at the social transformation of chronicity imposed as the main public health problems in force today and which make it difficult to engage in self-care (FORTALEZA, 2014).

Among the JCs (100.0%), there were contributions that expanded the relevance of CE and subsidised its incorporation into the monitoring of hypertensive patients in primary care, as follows:

- Description of the nursing intervention related to the ED "Risk of overweight" - refer to the nutritionist and/or the NASF, since not all NASFs have this professional.

The NASF is based on the dimensions of comprehensiveness, welcoming and humanised care, and is therefore a strategy that favours actions that integrate other social policies, such as those relating to education, sport, culture, work, leisure, etc. It is made up of a multi-professional team that works in partnership with ESF professionals, providing technical and pedagogical support to the teams in the units under its responsibility (SANTOS, 2012).

According to Ordinance 154 of 24 January 2008 in Art. 2 § 1, the NASF is not a gateway to the system, and must work in an integrated manner with the health services network, based on the demands identified in joint work with the ESF (BRASIL, 2017).

- Replacing the verb "to raise awareness" with "to sensitise".

To raise awareness means the feeling or knowledge that allows human beings to experience, experience or understand aspects or the totality of their inner world; the sense or perception that human beings have of what is morally right or wrong in individual acts and motives. And to sensitise means to make sensitive, impressionable, to provoke sensitisation.

Although the term "sensitising" was used by the nurses, awareness-raising is still the best health education strategy as it enables users not only to feel, but to know, experience, experiment and understand aspects related to their care.

- Updating ESF nurses on "EC" for implementation purposes.

ESF nurses should be trained regularly with updates on current guidelines and protocols, in line with the National Policy for Permanent Education in Health (PNEPS), which is based on meaningful learning and the possibility of transforming professional practices. Continuing education can be understood as work-based learning, i.e. it takes place in the daily lives of people and organisations (BRASIL, 2009).

- Nurse home visits to users using a family approach to the health/disease/treatment/rehabilitation process.

Home health care is a practice that dates back to the very existence of families as a unit of social organisation. It has emerged as an alternative to hospital care, provoking the possibility of reclaiming the home as a space for producing care and emerging as a device for producing the deinstitutionalisation of care and new technological arrangements for health work, bringing great potential for innovation (BRASIL, 2012).

Home care should provide for the family in their private and domestic social space, respecting the movement and complexity of family relationships. The health professional must have an attitude of respect and appreciation of the peculiar characteristics of that human conviviality, taking a comprehensive approach in the home setting because it involves multiple factors in the family's health-disease process, influencing the forms of care (BRASIL, 2012).

- Drawing up a letter to municipal, state and federal managers to publicise and incorporate EC into the ESF.

The continuous growth in health spending, the increasing production of new technologies and the changes in the epidemiological profile of populations over the last two decades have led to diversified care needs. This makes it socially and politically necessary to develop mechanisms to coordinate the sectors involved in the production, incorporation and use of technologies in health systems (BRASIL, 2010).

Current discussions on the impact of these policies consider that health knowledge is articulated from a population and social perspective, going beyond the limits of individual clinical practice. It is therefore necessary to make managers aware of the proposed EC, presenting it to them in printed and digital format, demonstrating the impact of the proposal on self-care for users with SAH.

CHAPTER 8

NURSING CONSULTATION - Educational technology for the self-care of people with hypertension

8.1 Presentation of the Nursing Consultation

The Nursing Consultation (NC) was based on the theoretical framework of Orem (1995). The NC contains five stages - data collection, diagnosis, planning, implementation and evolution/evaluation.

The following forms were used to carry out the NC: Data survey, which was drawn up by Santos and Silva (2002) already validated; Nursing Care Plan (NCP), with the Nursing Diagnoses (ND) based on the Taxonomy of the North American Nursing Diagnosis Association (NANDA 20152017) listed according to Orem's "Self-Care Requirements" (1995) with the respective interventions and expected results, based on NIC (Nursing Intevention Classification) and NOC (Nursing Outcomes Classification) (2012).

The EDs were selected a priori on the basis of the researcher's experiences of accompanying people with SAH, and were the most frequently identified.

The following instruments are available to carry out the NC: Data Survey; Nursing Care Plan (NCP); and Instructional Guide for the Nursing Consultation.

NURSING CONSULTATION - Health education technology for the self-care of people with hypertension

DATA COLLECTION[1]

I - Identification

Name _______________________________ UAPS <u>Date</u>___/___/___________

Record No. SUS Card No.

Age: Religion: Marital status:No. of children:

Place of birth: _____________________ Origin: _______________________________

Family income (minimum wages): _________ Level of education _____________________

Race/colour: ___ Housing conditions: _____________________Occupation: ______________

Address: ____

Who you live with ____

II - Universal Self-Care

1. Oxygenation (environmental and organic): ___________________________________

---

[1] SANTOS, Z.M.S.A.; SILVA, R.M. Hipertensão arterial: modelo de educação em saúde para o autocuidado. Fortaleza (CE): UNIFOR; 2002.

2. Hydration (types, routes, daily quantity and quality) ____

3. Nutrition (habits, preferences, taboos, intolerances, restrictions, allergies, changes) ______________________

4. Eliminations (intestinal, urinary, respiratory, gastric, other): _______________________________

5. Activity and rest (hours of activity and sleep per day, type, satisfaction and need for help to reconcile sleep): ____

6. Loneliness and social interaction (presence or absence of loneliness, participation in social activities, family and social relationships): ____

7. Risks to life and well-being (smoking, alcoholism, excessive use of coffee, use of hypertensive medication, stress, family history, dyslipidaemia, overweight/obesity and sedentary lifestyle)

____

____

____

8. health promotion (prevention of breast, cervical and prostate cancer, basic immunisation, six-monthly dental check-ups and annual ophthalmological check-ups): ____

III - "Developmental" self-care

1. Life cycle change(s): ____

Meaning of the changes: ____

2. Adaptation to change(s) (physical, psychological and social) _______________________________

3. Reproductive function (age at menarche, menstrual cycle, age and type of menopause, clinical manifestations of the climacteric, birth control, number of pregnancies, births and abortions)

____

____

____

4. Sexual activity (beginning and end, number of partners, frequency and aspect of relations, prevention and control of STD/AIDS and alterations)

____

____

____

IV - Self-care for Health Deviations

1. Discovery of the disease: ____

2. Diagnosis and treatment time: ____

3. Type(s) of treatment: ____

4. Knowledge of the disease and treatment: ____

5. Effective execution of the orientated behaviours: _________________________________

6. Existence of other health problems: ____

PHYSICAL EXAMINATION:

PA: __________   Member/Cir: __________   Position: __________
Wrist __________   FC: __________   FR: __________

                Height: __________
Weight: __________   IMC: __________
Head: ____

Neck: ____

Anterior trunk:

Chest: ____

Lungs: ____

Heart: ____

Breasts: ____

Armpits: ____

Abdomen: ____

Genitals: ____

Posterior trunk:

Back and spine: ____

Buttocks: ____

Anus and rectum: ____

Members:

Superiors: ____

Lower: ____

Hygiene conditions, personal appearance and clothing: ______________________________

Comments: ____

SELF-CARE ASSESSMENTS

CA demand(s) related to: ____

Capacity for CA: yes ( ) no ( ) partial ( )   total ( )

Nursing system(s): ____

Method(s) to help with self-care: ____

NURSING CARE PLAN

NAME: __________ UAPS__________DATE: _____ /___/

PRONTUÁRIO number__________ SUS CARD number__________

Self-care requirements[1]	Cd.DE	X	Diagnosis of Nursing (DE)[2]	X	Nursing Interventions (NIC)[3]	Results Expected (NOC)[4]
U - Adequate oxygenation	00180		Risk of contamination		Advising on the risks of atmospheric pollutants for individual, family and collective health Guidance on identifying atmospheric pollutants Raising awareness of the elimination and/or control of atmospheric pollutants Guidance on maintaining the hygiene of the environment	Knowledge of risk prevention and control.
	00181		Contamination related to exposure to atmospheric pollutants		Advising on the risks of atmospheric pollutants for individual, family and collective health Guidance on identifying atmospheric pollutants Raising awareness of the elimination and/or control of atmospheric pollutants Guidance on maintaining environmental hygiene and personal protection measures	Knowledge safety and security practices.
U- Nutrition Adequate	00232		Obesity related to poor eating behaviour		Advising on health risks Guidance on portioning daily meals Guidance on the predominance of white meat and vegetables in daily meals Referral to nutritionist and physical educator	Knowledge about proper diet.
	00233		Overweight related to poor eating behaviour		Advising on health risks Guidance on portioning daily meals Guidance on the predominance of white meat and vegetables in daily meals Referral to nutritionist and physical educator	Behaviour of adherence to the right diet, and weight loss and maintenance.
	00234		Risk of overweight		Identifying eating disorders Guidance on the health risks of weight gain Guidance on portioning daily meals Encouraging regular physical exercise	Knowledge about proper diet and weight control
	00179		Risk of unstable glycaemia		Guidance on treatment follow-up Raising awareness about the use of artificial sweeteners Encouraging regular physical exercise Raising awareness of the importance of following the Food Plan	Control of glycaemia and prevention of *diabetes mellitus*
Adequate hydration	00028		Risk of insufficient fluid volume		Guidance on adequate fluid intake and its health benefits. Encourage the daily intake of 1.5 to 2 liquids a day	Knowledge and adequate water intake
U-Suitable eliminations	00022		Risk of Urge Urinary Incontinence		Provide guidance on infection prevention measures. Guidance on pelvic muscle strengthening exercises	Knowledge about proper urinary elimination
	00011		Constipation related to poor eating habits, insufficient fluid intake and irregular bowel		Guidance on regular bowel habits. Encourage adequate water intake. Raising awareness of the importance of following the Food Plan Refer to nutritionist.	Knowledge about proper intestinal elimination

		movements		
	00015	Risk of constipation	Guidance on regular bowel habits. Encourage adequate water intake. Raising awareness about following the Food Plan Refer to nutritionist.	Knowledge about proper intestinal elimination
U-Activity balance and rest	00092	Activity intolerance related to a sedentary lifestyle	Guidance on regular physical exercise Guidance on body mechanics Ask for family support Guidance on an environment free of environmental barriers Refer to physical educator	Activity tolerance, locomotion and physical conditioning.
	00095	Insomnia related to frequent daytime naps and inadequate sleep hygiene	Teaching relaxation techniques (massages) Adopt a calm, comfortable and noise-free environment Investigate and eliminate or control the causes of insomnia Adopt regular sleep (night) and rest (day) schedules	Endurance and energy conservation. Adequate sleep and rest
	00088	Impaired ambulation related to impaired balance and vision	Guidance on seeking family support in carrying out essential activities of daily living (self-care) Guidance on stretching exercises, joint mobility and muscle strengthening	Locomotion- walking, balance, movement, co-ordination, endurance and mobility.
	00155	Risk of falls	Guidance on preventing falls Referral to Physiotherapist and Ophthalmologist Guidance on body mechanics Ask for family support Guidance on an environment free of environmental barriers	Performance of body mechanics, coordinated movement and mobility Rehabilitation therapy.
U- Balance between solitude and social interaction	00052	Impaired social interaction related to insufficient knowledge of how to strengthen reciprocity	Encouraging participation in recreational therapies (groups, lectures) Stimulate the maintenance of the family process Providing an environment for active and effective listening Investing in socialisation	Social interaction and involvement skills
	00054	Risk of loneliness	Carry out active and qualified listening to the person's demands Encourage family support in this socialisation process Refer to psychologist	Family well-being. Participation in leisure. Humour balance.
	00223	Ineffective relationships related to developmental crises	Promoting family integrity and involvement Encourage goal-setting Encouraging family and friend interaction	Development: stages of the life cycle. Role performance
	00053	Social isolation related to factors that impact on satisfactory	Encourage participation in recreational activities Encouraging socialisation and social skills Integrating the family into the health-disease	Involvement and Social support

		personal relationships	process Request psychological support if necessary	
U-Risk to life and Well-being	00048	Damaged teeth related to poor oral hygiene	- Guidance on the importance of oral hygiene after each meal - Referral to the Oral Health Team	Knowledge about oral hygiene. Motivation. Physical fitness. Energy conservation
	00168	Sedentary lifestyle related to poor knowledge	Encouraging regular physical exercise Guidance on the importance of regular physical exercise for health	Dietary guidance-reduction.
	00188	about the health benefits of physical activity. Risk-prone health behaviour related to low self-efficacy	Refer to physical educator Leading to self-responsibility for health Guidance on substance abuse with alcohol, cigarettes, etc. Encourage people to reduce their salt and fat intake. Encourage family involvement	Adherence of behaviour
	00043	Ineffective protection related to substance abuse and extremes of age	Guidance on identifying health risks Promoting health education to change behaviour	Healthy lifestyle
	00193	Self-neglect related to lifestyle choices	- Guidance on essential activities of daily living - Guidance on healthy lifestyle habits	
U-Health promotion	00099 00097	Ineffective health maintenance related to insufficient resources Poor recreational activity related to age extremes and insufficient reactive activities.	Promoting health education Improve support systems Advice on health services Providing guidance on health rights and duties Identify community health resources Refer to social services. Regular visits to the dentist, ophthalmologist, gynaecologist and urologist. Enquire about leisure options Referral to social groups Encouraging complementary and integrative practices Referral to occupational therapist	Access to care resources. Knowledge and behaviour and health promotion and health seeking. Social support. Acceptance behaviour, adherence, health orientation.
D-Adapting to changes in the life cycle	00065	Ineffective sexuality pattern related to insufficient knowledge of sexuality-related alternatives	Guidance on the changes that are relevant to the stage of the life cycle Promoting sexual counselling Promoting couples/group therapy Referral to a specialist doctor (Gynaecologist or Urologist)	Knowledge about physical ageing
	00133	Chronic pain related to female gender	Guidance on the potential appropriate to the life cycle Encouraging physical exercise Adopt therapeutic and comfortable positions	Pain control. Adapting to
			- Refer to a doctor.	changes in the life cycle
D-Social adaptation	00014 6	Anxiety related to conflict over life goals	Encouraging new activities Discuss life goal strategies Providing emotional and decision-making	Self-control of anxiety Concentration

	00069	Ineffective coping related to ineffective resources	support Referral to psychologist and occupational therapist Providing spiritual and emotional support Referral for psychological assessment Stimulate improvement in body self-image Encourage improved self-esteem and self-perception	Personal resilience Self-esteem Psychosocial adaptation
	00177	Stress overload related to insufficient resources	Guidance on monitoring activities of daily living Providing social support Elect a family member to make decisions Discuss access to resources in the community	Personal well-being Self-esteem Social support
DS-Knowledge about the disease	00126	Poor knowledge related to insufficient information	Encourage teaching techniques about the disease process Providing memory training Guidance on hypertension	Knowledge about hypertension.
DS-Knowledge about the treatment	00161	Poor knowledge related to insufficient information	Guidance on how to control the disease Raising awareness of the importance of the therapeutic plan Defining the health and disease process - Clarify doubts and errors that may arise	Knowledge of hypertension control
DS-Acceptance of the disease	00121	Disturbed personal identity related to situational crisis	Ask for psychosocial support in coping with decision-making Promoting family involvement in the health-disease process Assess possible threat situations	Confrontation. Decision-making Acceptance of chronicity
DS-Adaptation to illness and treatment	00125	Feeling of powerlessness related to complex treatment regime	Periodic referral for psychological assessment Inform about the importance of following the proposed therapeutic plan Carry out active and qualified listening whenever necessary Encouraging lifestyle adaptation to treatment	Health beliefs: perception of performance capacity, perception of control and resources. State of comfort Participation in healthcare decisions Personal autonomy
	00214	Impaired comfort related to treatment regime	Ask about the possible discomforts of the treatment Guidance on how to control the disease Informing about the health commitment in order to promote better situational control	
DS-Effective execution of orientated behaviours	00079	Lack of adherence related to inadequate access to care, prolonged duration of the regime, and insufficient knowledge about the regime	Providing easy access to the health system for individuals and their families Promote the continuity of the proposed therapeutic process Provide sufficient social support Establish a treatment regime compatible with each person Guidance on the proposed therapeutic plan/regimen Elect a family member as a carer Encourage the inclusion of the treatment regime in daily life	Carer performance: direct and indirect care Adherence behaviour. Motivation Family functioning

2015-2017 (NANDA International). Organisers: HERDMAN, T.H; KAMITSURU, S. Translation: GARCEZ, R. M. Technical review: BARROS, A. L. B.L *et al.* Porto Alegre: Artmed; 2015. 468p)

[3,4]JOHNSON, M *et al.* NANDA - NOC-NIC linkages: clinical conditions - supporting critical reasoning and quality care. 3 ed. (Translation of NOC and NIC Linkages to NANDA -I and Clinical Conditions - Supporting Critical Reasoning and Quality Care, 3rd.ed; by Soraya Imon de Oliveira *et al*). Rio de Janeiro: Elsevier; 2012.

CHAPTER 9

CONCLUSIONS AND RECOMMENDATIONS

Analysing the results shows that the proposed EC was validated by the judges as a strategy for engaging people with SAH in self-care, as a complete and complex technology, relevant to the user, the nurse, the professional category and the institution.

The proposed EC contemplates all the self-care requirements proposed by Orem (1995), enabling nurses to lead hypertensive people to engage in self-care in order to maintain their health.

The incorporation of EC into the health system will certainly require both facilities and difficulties or resistance, such as time to apply the instruments, training for nurses on the subject, and making the material available in electronic format to make it easier to handle and record the interventions, as well as periodic monitoring of the proposed self-care on a monthly basis. To this end, the collaboration of the actors involved in health care - managers and nurses - will be essential.

It should be emphasised that the JTs resisted answering the data collection instrument, as it took several face-to-face contacts. This fact reflects the insipience or even lack of relevance given by nurses to CE. Therefore, it is opportune to explore this theme in nurse training institutions, as well as the involvement of professional bodies in incorporating SC into nurses' professional practice in the various care scenarios. However, innovative thinking in nursing is necessary for co-participation between the subjects involved in the teaching-learning process and recognising the diversity of knowledge as an enriching aspect of teaching.

Thus, nurses need to understand that care and technology are interlinked, because nursing is committed to principles, laws and theories and that technology consists of the expression of this scientific knowledge and its own transformation as a science, making the professional reflect critically and participatively on their being, with EC being a systematic, scientifically structured practice, with a unique language, in order to favour the promotion, protection and maintenance of life, favouring the self-care of hypertensive users, their families and the community.

The results of this study will be presented to the Nursing Managers and Coordinators at the UAPS for dissemination and later implementation (in printed and/or digital format) with the aim of instrumentalising the work of nurses, as health educators, in engaging users in self-care to control SAH and maintain their health in general, extending the preventive actions of this condition to family members, consequently minimising the problem of SAH for Public Health, which will expand with the predominance of elderly people in the Brazilian population.

REFERENCES

ALENCAR, Delmo de Carvalho et al. Nursing consultation from the perspective of users with diabetes mellitus in the Family Health Strategy. **Rev. Enferm. UFPE on line**, v. 11, n. 10, p. 37493756, 2017. Disponívelem:<http://bases.bireme.br/cgi-bin/wxislind.exe/iah/online/?IsisScript=iah/iah.xis&src=google&base=BDENF&lang=p&nextActio n=lnk&exprSearch=33046&indexSearch=ID>.

ARAUJO, Caroline Barão et al. The practice of self-care by nursing workers in basic health units. **Revista Eletrônica de Enfermagem**, v. 18, 2016. Available at: <https://www.revistas.ufg.br/fen/article/view/39304>.

ARAÚJO, Gilmara Barboza da Silva; GARCIA, Telma Ribeiro. Adherence to anti-hypertensive treatment: a conceptual analysis. **Rev. Eletrônica Enferm**, v. 8, n. 2, p. 259-272, 2006. Available at: <http://bases.bireme.br/cgi-bin/wxislind.exe/iah/online/?IsisScript=iah/iah.xis&src=google&base=BDENF&lang=p&nextActio n=lnk&exprSearch=13831&indexSearch=ID>.

BARBIANI, Rosangela; NORA, Carlise Rigon Dalla; SCHAEFER, Rafaela. Nursing practices in the primary health care context: a scoping review. **Revista latino-americana de enfermagem**, v. 24, 2016. Availablefrom:<http://www.scielo.br/scielo.php?pid=S0104-11692016000100609&script=sci_arttext&tlng=es>.

BARRETO, Mayckel da Silva et al. Non-utilisation of routine consultations in Primary Care by people with hypertension. **Ciência & Saúde Coletiva**, v. 23, p. 795-804, 2018. Available at: <https://www.scielosp.org/scielo.php?script=sci_arttext&pid=S1413-81232018000300795>.

BARROSO, Léa Maria Moura et al. Usefulness of the self-care theory in assisting patients with the Human Immunodeficiency Virus/Acquired Immunodeficiency Syndrome. **Acta Paulista de Enfermagem**, v. 23, n. 4, p. 562-567, 2010. Available at: <http://www.redalyc.org/html/3070/307023863019/>.

BELLINGER, Gene; CASSTRO, Durval; MILLS, Anthony. **Date, Information, Knowledge, and Wisdom**. Accessed 11/15/02. Available from:<http://www.outsights.com/systems/dikw/dikw.htm>

BRANDÃO, A. A.; AMODEO, C., NOBRE, F. **Hipertensão.** 2. ed., p. 511, Rio de Janeiro: Elsevier, 2012.

BRAZIL. Federal Council of Nursing. Resolution no. 0544/2017. Provides for Nursing Consultation. Brasília-DF, 9 May 2017.

______ . Ministry of Health. **Carta dos Direitos dos Usuários da Saúde**. 2 ed. Brasília: Ministério da Saúde, 2007.

. Ministry of Health. Ordinance No. 2,436, of 21 September 2017. Approves the National Primary Care Policy, establishing revised guidelines for the organisation of Primary Care, within the scope of the Unified Health System (SUS). Brasília: Ministry of Health, 2017.

______ . Ministry of Health. Health Care Secretariat. Department of Primary Care. **Home care booklet.** Brasília: Ministry of Health, 2012.

______ . Ministry of Health. Health Care Secretariat. **PNH - National Humanisation Policy.** Brasília: Ministry of Health, 2013.

______ . Ministry of Health. Health Care Secretariat. **National Primary Care Policy.** Brasília: Ministry of Health, 2017.

______ . Ministry of Health. Secretariat of Science, Technology and Strategic Inputs. Department of Science and Technology. **National Health Technology Management Policy**. Brasília: Ministry of Health, 2010.

______ . Ministry of Health. Secretariat for Labour Management and Health Education. Department of Health Education Management. **National Policy for Permanent Education in Health.** Brasília: Ministry of Health, 2009.

______ . Ministry of Health. Department of Health Situation Analysis. **Saúde Brasil 2006: an analysis of the health situation in Brazil.** Brasília: Ministry of Health; 2006.

______ . Ministry of Health. Health Surveillance Secretariat. Health Care Secretariat. **National Health Promotion Policy**. 3 ed., Brasília: Ministry of Health, 2010.

BULLINGER, M. et al. Developing and evaluating cross-cultural instruments from minimum requirements to optimal models. **Quality of Life Research**, v. 2, n. 6, p. 451-459, 1993. Available from: <https://link.springer.com/article/10.1007/BF00422219>.

BURRELL, Lisa Anne. Integrating critical thinking strategies into nursing curricula. **Teaching and Learning in Nursing,** v. 9, n. 2, p. 53-58, 2014. Available from: <https://www.sciencedirect.com/science/article/pii/S155730871300142X>.

CAMPEDELLI, Maria Coeli et al... **Processo de enfermagem na prática**. 2 ed. São Paulo: Ática, 2000.

CAMPOS, Célia Maria Sivalli; MISHIMA, Silvana Martins. Health needs through the voice of civil society and the State. **Cadernos de Saúde Pública,** v. 21, p. 1260-1268, 2005. Available at: <https://www.scielosp.org/scielo.php?script=sci_arttext&pid=S0102-311X2005000400029>.

CARPESITO, M. **Manual of nursing diagnoses**. 11. ed. Porto Alegre: Artmed, 2016.

CARVALHO, Ana Luiza Santos et al. Evaluation of nursing consultation records in gynaecology. **Revista Eletrônica de Enfermagem,** v. 10, n. 2, p.472-83, 2008. Available at: <http://fen.ufg.br/fen_revista/v10/n2/pdf/v10n2a18.pdf>.

CAVALCANTI, Ana Carla Dantas; CORREIA, Dayse Mary da Silva; QUELUCI, Gisella de Carvalho. The implementation of the nursing consultation for patients with heart failure. **Revista Eletrônica de Enfermagem,** v. 11, n. 1, p.103-104, 2009. Available at: <https://www.revistas.ufg.br/fen/article/view/46920>.

CHERNICHARO, Isis de Moraes. **The elderly in the contemporary world and new technologies.** 2018. 131f. Thesis (Doctorate in Nursing) - CHERNICHARO, Isis de Moraes. The elderly in the contemporary world and new technologies. Rio de Janeiro, 2018.

CHIANCA, T. C. M. The classifications of nursing practice: diagnoses, interventions and results. In: **III Forum Mineiro de Enfermagem:** Sistematizar o Cuidado, 2002. Uberlândia: Rápida Editora, 2002. v. 3. p. 50-66.

COFEN. Federal Nursing Council. Resolution 358/2009. Provides for the Systematisation of Nursing Care and the implementation of the Nursing Process in environments, public or private, in which professional nursing care takes place, and makes other provisions. Brasília-DF, 15 October 2009.

COSTA, Fernanda et al. Alternative inactivated poliovirus vaccines adjuvanted with Quillaja brasiliensis or Quil-A saponins are equally effective in inducing specific immune responses. **PloS one,** v. 9, n. 8, p. e105374,

2014. Available from:
<https://journals.plos.org/plosone/article?id=10.1371/journal.pone.0105374>.

CRAVEN, Ruth F.; HIRNLE, Constance. **Fundamentals of Nursing:** Human Health and Function. 4. ed. Rio de Janeiro: Guanabara Koogan S.A., 2006. 1492 p.

DANTAS, Cilene Nunes; SANTOS, Viviane Euzébia Pereira; TOURINHO, Francis Solange Vieira. The nursing consultation as a technology of care in the light of the thoughts of Bacon and Galimberti. **Texto &Contexto-Enfermagem,** v. 25, n. 1, 2016. Available at: <http://www.scielo.br/scielo.php?pid=S0104-07072016000100601&script=sci_abstract&tlng=es>.
DOCHTERMAN, J.M.; BULECCHECK, G.K.; **Classifications of nursing interventions (NIC).** 4. ed., Porto Alegre: Artmed, 2014. p. 988

DOMINGOS, Camila Santana et al. Construction and content validation of the nursing history guided by the orem reference. **Revista Mineira de Enfermagem,** v. 19, n. 2, p. 165-186, 2015. Available at: <http://www.reme.org.br/artigo/detalhes/1013>.

DOTTO, Jéssica Ineu et al. Systematisation of nursing care: order, disorder or (re)organisation? **Rev. Enferm. UFPE on line,** v. 11, n. 10, p. 3821-3829, 2017. Available at: <http://bases.bireme.br/cgibin/wxislind.exe/iah/online/?IsisScript=iah/iah.xis&src=google&base=B DENF&lang=p&nextAction=lnk&exprSearch=33055&indexSearch=ID>.

ENGELA, Maria Helena Trindade et al. Use of health technologies in primary care for people with systemic arterial hypertension. **Rev. Pesqui. Cuid. (Online),** v. 10, n. 1, p. 75-84, 2018. Available at:<http://bases.bireme.br/cgi-bin/wxislind.exe/iah/online/?IsisScript=iah/iah.xis&src=google&base=BDENF&lang=p&nextActio n=lnk&exprSearch=32258&indexSearch=ID>.

FEENBERG, Andrew. Technology and human finitude. **Revista de Filosofia Aurora,** v. 27, n. 40, p. 245-261, 2015. Available from: <https://periodicos.pucpr.br/index.php/aurora/article/view/676>.

FERNANDES, Helen Nicoletti et al. Interpersonal relationship in the work of the multiprofessional team of a family health unit. **Revista de Pesquisa Cuidado é Fundamental Online,** v. 7, n. 1, p.1915-1926 , 2015. Available at: <http://www.redalyc.org/html/5057/505750945016/>.

FERREIRA, Ana Clara Trindade et al. Childcare consultation: challenges and perspectives for nursing care for children and their families. **Revista Vivências**, v. 11, n. 20, p.231-241, 2015. Available at: <http://www.reitoria.uri.br/~vivencias/Numero_020/artigos/pdf/Artigo_19.pdf>.

FLORES, Cezar Augusto da Silva; ALMEIDA, Patrícia Bilha de; MARTINI JUNIOR, Ercílio. Investigation and Historical Documentation of Nursing in the Northern Region of the State of Mato Grosso - Brazil. **Hist. enferm., Rev. eletronica**, v. 8, n. 1, p. 18-26, 2017. Available at: <http://bases.bireme.br/cgi-bin/wxislind.exe/iah/online/?IsisScript=iah/iah.xis&src=google&base=BDENF&lang=p&nextActio n=lnk&exprSearch=32306&indexSearch=ID>.

FLORES, Giovana Ely; OLIVEIRA, Dora Lúcia Leidens Corrêa de; ZOCCHE, Denise Antunes de Azambuja. Continuing education in the hospital context: an experience that gives new meaning to nursing care. **Trabalho, educação & saúde**, v. 14, n. 2, p. 487-504, 2016. Available at: <https://www.lume.ufrgs.br/handle/10183/142545>.

FREIRE, P.; **Pedagogy of the oppressed.** São Paulo: Paz e Terra, 2001.

GARCIA, Telma Ribeiro. Systematisation of nursing care: a substantive aspect of professional practice. **Anna Nery School of Nursing Journal**, v. 20, n. 1, p. 5-6, 2016. Available at: <http://www.redalyc.org/pdf/1277/127744318001.pdf>.

GERARD, Sally O. et al. Past, present, and future trends of master's education in nursing. **Journal of Professional Nursing**, v. 30, n. 4, p. 326-332, 2014. Available from: <https://www.sciencedirect.com/science/article/pii/S8755722314000337>.

GOMES, Andréa Tayse de Lima et al. Technologies applied to patient safety: a bibliometric review. **Revista de Enfermagem do Centro-Oeste Mineiro**, v. 7, p.1473, 2017. Available at: <http://www.seer.ufsj.edu.br/index.php/recom/article/view/1473>.

GOMES, Iago Vieira et al. Characterisation of hypertensive users treated at a 24-hour emergency care unit. **Nursing**, v. 21, n. 239, p. 2114-2118, 2018. Available at: <http://bases.bireme.br/cgibin/wxislind.exe/iah/online/?IsisScript=iah/iah.xis&src=google&base=B DENF&lang=p&nextAction=lnk&exprSearch=32914&indexSearch=ID>.

JAMES, Paul A. et al. 2014 evidence-based guideline for the management of high blood pressure in adults:

report from the panel members appointed to the Eighth Joint National Committee (JNC 8). **Jama,** v. 311, n. 5, p. 507-520, 2014. Available from: <https://jamanetwork.com/journals/jama/fullarticle/1791497>.

JOHNSON, M.; MAAS, M.; MOORHEAD, S. **Nursing Outcomes Classification (NOC).** 2. ed., Porto Alegre: Artmed, 2014.

JOHNSON, Marion et al. **NANDA - NOC - NIC links: clinical conditions:** support for reasoning and quality care. Rio de Janeiro: Elsevier, 2012.

KELLY, K. **Where technology is taking us.** Porto Alegre: Bookman, 2012.

KLAFKE, Andre; VAGHETTI, Laura Afanador Pineros; COSTA, Andre Dias. Effect of attachment to a family doctor on blood pressure control in hypertensive patients. **Revista Brasileira de Medicina de Família e Comunidade,** v. 12, n. 39, p. 1-7, 2017. Available at: <https://rbmfc.emnuvens.com.br/rbmfc/article/view/1444>.

LAING, R. D.; PHILLIPSON, H.; LEE, A. R. **Interpersonal Perception:** a theory and a research method. Rio de Janeiro: Eldorado; 2016.

LEIDY, Yadira et al. Social-scientific issues and moral and ethical reasoning. **TED: Tecné, Episteme y Didaxis, n. Extra,** p. 8-21, 2014. Addtional: <http://revistas.pedagogica.edu.co/index.php/TED/article/view/3184>.

LEVY, P. **The technologies of intelligence.** Rio de Janeiro: Editora 34, 2016.

LIMA, Juliana Vieira Figueiredo et al. Usefulness of comfort theory for clinical nursing care for puerperal women: critical analysis. **Revista Gaúcha de Enfermagem,** v. 37, n. 4, 2016. Available at:<http://www.scielo.br/scielo.php?pid=S1983-14472016000400701&script=sci_abstract&tlng=es>.

LOPES, Emeline Moura et al. Self-care theory in the care of women living with AIDS: usefulness of the theory. **Rev. Av. Enferm.** v.33, n.2, p.241-250, 2015. Available at: <http://www.scielo.org.co/pdf/aven/v33n2/v33n2a06.pdf>.

LORENZETTI, Jorge et al. Technology, technological innovation and health: a necessary reflection. **Texto & Contexto Enfermagem**, v. 21, n. 2,   2012. Available at: <http://www.redalyc.org/html/714/71422962023/>.

LYNN, Mary R. Determination and quantification of content validity. **Nursing research**, v. 35, n. 6, p. 382-385, 1986. Available from: <https://insights.ovid.com/crossref?an=00006199-198611000- 00017>.

MACIEL, Isabel Cristina Filgueira; DE ARAÚJO, Thelma Leite. Nursing consultation: analysis of actions in hypertension programmes in Fortaleza. **Revista Latino-Americana de Enfermagem**,   v. 11, n. 2, p. 207-214,   2003. Available at: <http://www.scielo.br/pdf/rlae/v11n2/v11n2a10>.

MALACHIAS, M. V. B. et *al*. 7ª Brazilian hypertension guideline. **Arq Bras Cardiol**, v. 107, n. 3, p. 1-103, 2016. Available at: <http://publicacoes.cardiol.br/2014/diretrizes/2016/05_HIPERTENSAO_ARTERIAL.pdf>.

MALTA, Deborah Carvalho et al. Health care in adults with self-reported hypertension in Brazil according to data from the National Health Survey, 2013. **Revista Brasileira de Epidemiologia**, v. 18, p. 109-122, 2015. Available at: <https://www.scielosp.org/scielo.php?pid=S1415-790X2015000700109&script=sci_arttext>.

MALTA, Deborah Carvalho; SILVA JR, Jarbas Barbosa da. The Strategic Action Plan for Tackling Chronic Non-Communicable Diseases in Brazil and the definition of global targets for tackling these diseases by 2025: a review. **Epidemiologia e Serviços de Saúde**, v. 22, n. 1, p. 151-164, 2013. Available at: <http://scielo.iec.gov.br/scielo.php?lng=pt&pid=S1679- 49742013000100016&script=sci_arttext>.

MARIOSA, Duarcides Ferreira; FERRAZ, Renato Ribeiro Nogueira; SANTOS-SILVA, Edinaldo Nelson dos. Influence of socio-environmental conditions on the prevalence of systemic arterial hypertension in two riverside communities in the Amazon, Brazil. **Ciência & Saúde Coletiva**, v. 23, p. 14251436, 2018. Available at: <https://www.scielosp.org/scielo.php?script=sci_arttext&pid=S1413- 81232018000501425>.

MARTINS, Rafael da Silva Tavares; NASCIMENTO, Deyvison Roberto. Industrialisation as an agent for transforming quality of life. **Revista Univap**, v. 22, n. 40, p. 51, 2016. Available at: <https://revista.univap.br/index.php/revistaunivap/article/view/1351>.

MOURA, Fabiana Maria; DA SILVA, Maria da Conceição Gomes; CARNUT, Leonardo. Cardiovascular Care Policy within the Unified Health System: brief comments on the available indexed scientific literature. **JMPHC-Journal of Management & Primary Health Care**, v. 2, n. 1, p. 30-33, 2011. Available at: <http://www.jmphc.com.br/jmphc/article/view/97>.

NANDA. **NANDA nursing diagnoses** - definitions and classifications 2015-2017. Organisers: HERDMAN, T.H; KAMITSURU, S. Translation: GARCEZ, R. M. Technical review: BARROS, A. L. B.L et al..Porto Alegre: Artmed, 2015.

OREM, D. **Nursing concepts of practice**. 5. ed. St Louis: Mosby Year Book, 1995.

PADILHA, Maria Itayra Coelho de Souza; BORENSTEIN, Miriam Susskind. The historical research method in nursing. **Texto & Contexto Enfermagem**, v. 14, n. 4, p.575-84, 2005. Available at: <http://www.index-f.com/textocontexto/2005pdf/2005-575.pdf>.

PEREIRA, Raliane Talita Alberto; FERREIRA, Viviane. The nursing consultation in the family health strategy. **Revista Brasileira Multidisciplinar**, v. 17, n. 1, p. 99-111, 2014. Available at: <http://www.revistarebram.com/index.php/revistauniara/article/view/10>.

PINHEIRO, R. **Everyday practices in the relationship between supply and demand of health services:** a field of study and construction of integrality. Rio de Janeiro: Abrasco, 2016. p.65-112

PINTO, Eliangela Saraiva Oliveira; RODRIGUES, Weliton Nepomuceno. Systematisation of Nursing Care in Primary Care for people with hypertension. **Nursing**, v. 21, n. 237, p. 2036-2040, 2018. Available at: <http://bases.bireme.br/cgi-bin/wxislind.exe/iah/online/?IsisScript=iah/iah.xis&src=google&base=BDENF&lang=p&nextActio n=lnk&exprSearch=32628&indexSearch=ID>.

PIRES, Denise Elvira Pires et al. Technological innovation and workloads of health professionals: an ambiguous relationship. **Revista Gaúcha de Enfermagem**, v. 33, n. 1, p. 157-168, 2012. Available at: <http://www.seer.ufrgs.br/RevistaGauchadeEnfermagem/article/view/20617>.

POLIT, Denise F. et al. **Fundamentals of nursing research:** methods, evaluation and utilisation. 5. ed. Porto Alegre: Artmed, 2011.

RÊGO, Anderson da Silva et al. Factors associated with inadequate blood pressure in people with hypertension. **Cogitare Enferm,** v. 23, n. 1, 2018. Available at: <https://revistas.ufpr.br/cogitare/article/view/54087>.

RODRIGUES, Cláudia Cristiane Filgueira Martins et al. Innovative nursing teaching from the perspective of epistemologies of the South. **Escola Anna Nery,** v. 20, n. 2, p. 384-389, 2016. Available at:<http://www.scielo.br/scielo.php?pid=S1414-81452016000200384&script=sci_abstract&tlng=es>.

ROLIM, Laurie Penha et al. Interaction between diabetes mellitus and hypertension on hearing in the elderly. **CoDAS. Sociedade Brasileira de Fonoaudiologia,** v. 27, n. 5, p. 428-432, 2015. Available at: <http://observatorio.fm.usp.br/handle/OPI/14639>.

SANTANA, Fabiana Ribeiro et al. Health actions in the family health strategy in the municipality of Goiás from the perspective of integrality. **Revista Eletronica de Enfermagem,** v. 15, n. 2, p.422-9, 2013. Available at: <http://projetos.extras.ufg.br/fen_revista/v15/n2/pdf/v15n2a15.pdf>.

SANTOS, R. C. **Saúde todo dia:** uma construção coletiva. São Paulo: Hucitec, 2017.

______ . The **Family Health Support Centre (NASF) as a component of mental health care:** perspectives of family health strategy professionals. 2012. 175 f. Dissertation (Master's in Public Health) - Federal University of Ceará. Faculty of Medicine, Fortaleza, 2012.

SANTOS, Z. M. S. A.; SILVA, R. M. **Hipertensão arterial:** modelo de educação em saúde para o autocuidado. Fortaleza (CE): UNIFOR; 2002.

SCHMITZ, Eudinéia Luz et al. Philosophy and conceptual framework: collectively structuring the systematisation of nursing care. **Revista Gaúcha de Enfermagem,** v. 37, n. spe, 2016. Available at:<http://www.scielo.br/scielo.php?pid=S1983-14472016000500405&script=sci_abstract&tlng=es>.

SECCO, Ana Caroline; PARABONI, Patrícia; ARPINI, Dorian Mônica. Groups as a care device in primary care for working with diabetics and hypertensive patients. **Mudanças-Psicologia da Saúde,** v. 25, n. 1, p. 9-15, 2017. Available at: <https://www.metodista.br/revistas/revistas-metodista/index.php/MUD/article/view/7355>.

SILVA, Josilaine Porfírio; GARANHANI, Mara Lucia; GUARIENTE, Maria Helena Dantas de Menezes.

Systematisation of nursing care and complex thinking in nurse training: a documentary analysis. **Revista Gaúcha de Enfermagem**, v. 35, n. 2, p. 128-134, 2014. Available at: <http://www.seer.ufrgs.br/RevistaGauchadeEnfermagem/article/view/44538>.

SILVA, Kênia Lara; SENA, Roseni Rosângela. Comprehensive health care: indications from nurse training. **Revista da Escola de Enfermagem da USP**, v. 42, n. 1, p. 48-56, 2008. Available at: <http://www.scielo.br/pdf/reeusp/v42n1/07>.

SILVA, Rafael Celestino da; FERREIRA, Márcia de Assunção. Technology in nursing care: an analysis based on the conceptual framework of Fundamental Nursing. **Revista Brasileira de Enfermagem**, v. 67, n. 1, p. 111-8, 2014. Available at: <http://www.redalyc.org/html/2670/267030130015/>.

SILVA, S.A.; BAITELO, T.C.; FRACOLLI, L.A. Avaliação da Atenção Primária a Saúde: a visão de usuários e profissionais sobre a estratégia de saúde da família. **Revista Latino Americana Enferm**, v.23, n.5, p.979-87, Sep/Oct, 2015.

SILVEIRA, Nalin Ferreira; VALMORBIDA, Willian. Labelling process for the implementation of RFID technology in the Univates University Centre Library. **RDBCI: Digital Journal of Library and Information Science**, v. 14, n. 2, p. 334-347, 2016. Available at: <https://periodicos.sbu.unicamp.br/ojs/index.php/rdbci/article/view/8641634>.

BRAZILIAN SOCIETY OF CARDIOLOGY. VI Brazilian hypertension guidelines. **Revista Bras Hipertens**, v. 17, n.1, p. 7-10, 2016.

SOUZA, A. P. M. A. et al. Implementation of Care: fourth phase of the nursing process. In: NÓBREGA, Maria Miriam Lima da; SILVA, Kenya de Lima (Org.). **Fundamentals of nursing care**. Belo Horizonte: Aben, 2016.

SOUZA, Ana Célia Caetano; MOREIRA, Thereza Maria Magalhães; BORGES, José Wicto Pereira. Educational technologies developed to promote cardiovascular health in adults: an integrative review. **Revista da Escola de Enfermagem da USP**, v. 48, n. 5, p. 944-951, 2014. Available at: <http://www.periodicos.usp.br/reeusp/article/view/103095>.

SOUZA, Elisangela et al. Health education for people with hypertension and diabetes in primary care. **Nursing**, v. 21, n. 240, p. 2178-2183, 2018. Available at: <http://bases.bireme.br/cgi-

bin/wxislind.exe/iah/online/?IsisScript=iah/iah.xis&src=google&base=BDENF&lang=p&nextActio
n=lnk&exprSearch=33088&indexSearch=ID>.

SOUZA, Rosana Santana de et al. Child health care: practices of Family Health nurses. **Revista Mineia de Enfermagem**, v. 17, n. 2, p. 331-348, 2013. Available at: <http://www.reme.org.br/artigo/detalhes/653>.

TANNURE, M. C.; PINHEIRO, A. M. **SAE:** Systematisation of nursing care: A PRACTICAL GUIDE. 2. ed. Rio de Janeiro: Guanabara Koogan, 2011.

TANNURE, Meire Chucre. **Bank of special nursing language terms for adult intensive care units.** 2008. 94f. Dissertation (Master's in Nursing) - Federal University of Minas Gerais, Belo Horizonte, 2008.

TAVARES, Marília Matias Kestering; SOUZA, Samara Tomé Correa. The elderly and barriers to accessing new information and communication technologies. **RENOTE**, v. 10, n. 1, 2012, p. 1-7, july 2012. Available at: <http://www.seer.ufrgs.br/renote/article/view/30915>.

TESTONI, Elen Ferraz et al. Nursing consultation and cardiometabolic control of diabetics: randomised clinical trial. **Rev Bras Enferm [Internet]**, v. 70, n. 3, p. 492-8, 2017. Available at: <https://www.researchgate.net/profile/Guilherme_Arruda/publication/317289290_Nursing_appoint ment_and_cardiometabolic_control_of_diabetics_a_randomised_clinical_trial/links/593c0d6fa6fdc c17a9e4ed44/Nursing-appointment-and-cardiometabolic-control-of-diabetics-a-randomised- clinical- trial.pdf>.

TRENTINI, Mercedes; GONÇALVES, Lucia Hisako Takase. Small convergence groups: a method for developing technologies in nursing. **Texto Contexto Enferm**, v. 9, n. 1, p. 63-78, 2000.

VITOR, Allyne Fortes; LOPES, Marcos Venícios de Oliveira; ARAUJO, Thelma Leite de. Teoria do déficit de autocuidado: análise da sua importância e aplicabilidade na prática de enfermagem. **Esc. Anna Nery**, Rio de Janeiro, v. 14, n. 3, p. 611-616, 2010. Available at: <http://www.scielo.br/pdf/ean/v14n3/v14n3a25>.

WEBER, Michael A. et al. Clinical practice guidelines for the management of hypertension in the community: a statement by the American Society of Hypertension and the International Society of Hypertension. **The journal of clinical hypertension**, v. 16, n. 1, p. 14-26, 2014. Available from: <https://onlinelibrary.wiley.com/doi/abs/10.1111/jch.12237>.

XAVIER, Lucélia Ferreira et al. Systematisation of nursing care: the knowledge of nurses in the municipality of JI-Paraná, Rondônia, Brazil. **Nursing**, v. 21, n. 239, p. 2110-2113, 2018. Available at:<http://bases.bireme.br/cgi-bin/wxislind.exe/iah/online/?IsisScript=iah/iah.xis&src=google&base=BDENF&lang=p&nextActio n=lnk&exprSearch=32913&indexSearch=ID>.

ZANGIROLANI, Lia Thieme Oikawa et al. Self-reported hypertension in adults living in Campinas, São Paulo, Brazil: prevalence, associated factors and control practices in a population-based study. **Ciência & Saúde Coletiva**, v. 23, p. 1221-1232, 2018. Available from: <https://www.scielosp.org/scielo.php?pid=S1413- 81232018000401221&script=sci_arttext&tlng=en>.

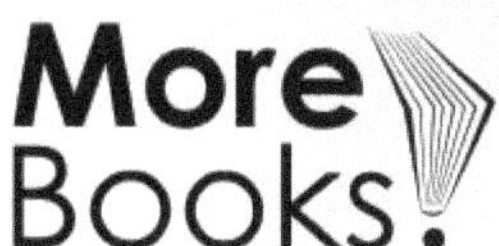

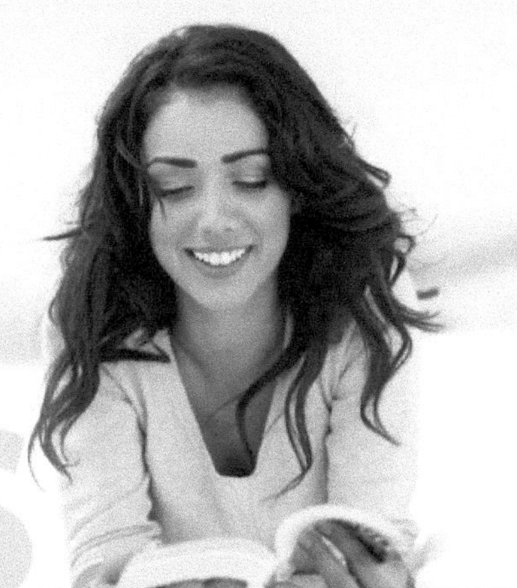

yes I want morebooks!

Buy your books fast and straightforward online - at one of world's fastest growing online book stores! Environmentally sound due to Print-on-Demand technologies.

Buy your books online at
www.morebooks.shop

Kaufen Sie Ihre Bücher schnell und unkompliziert online – auf einer der am schnellsten wachsenden Buchhandelsplattformen weltweit! Dank Print-On-Demand umwelt- und ressourcenschonend produziert.

Bücher schneller online kaufen
www.morebooks.shop

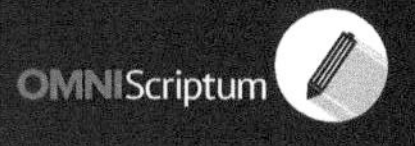

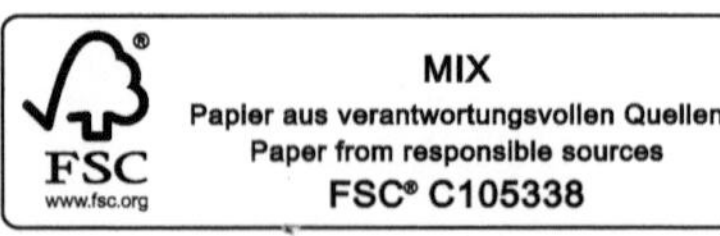

Printed by Books on Demand GmbH, Norderstedt / Germany